HABITS RULE YOU

One Simple Answer
to Achieving Your Nutrition & Fitness Goals

Angelica Ganea

HABITS RULE YOU: One Simple Answer to Achieving Your Nutrition & Fitness Goals
Copyright © 2017 by Angelica Ganea

All rights reserved. Without limiting the rights under the copyright reserved above, no part of this publication may be reproduced, stored in or introduced into a retrieval system, or transmitted in any form or by any means (electronic, mechanical, photocopying, recording or otherwise, without the prior written permission of the copyright owner.

DISCLAIMER: This publication contains the opinions and ideas of its author and is intended to provide advice concerning the subject matter covered. It is sold with the understanding that the author is not engaged in providing health, phychological or other professional services in this publication. This publication is not intended to provide a basis for action in particular circumstances without consideration by a competent professional. The author specifically disclaims any responsibility for any liability, loss or risk, personal or otherwise, that is incurred as a consequence, directly or indirectly, of the use and application of any of the contents of this book.

ISBN (Paperback): 978-0-9784940-2-5
ISBN (Hardcover): 978-0-9784940-3-2
ISBN (eBook): 978-0-9784940-4-9

www.HabitsRuleYou.com
www.AngelicaGanea.coom
info@AngelicaGanea.com

*"We are what we repeatedly do.
Excellence, then, is not an act, but a habit."*
— Aristotle

Contents

Acknowledgements xi
Introduction 1
Why Nutrition and Fitness? 11
Habits– Good *and* Bad– Rule Us 15
Give Simplicity A Chance 24

Part One: the Theory

Chapter 1: HOW LONG DOES IT TAKE TO FORM A HABIT? ... 35
    The Brain— Amygdala and Neural Pathways 41
    The Beliefs— Habits of Thought 54
    The Reward— *"What's In It For Me?!"* 65
    The Will— Your Habit Predecessor 78
    The Knowing— Know Who You Are and Where You Come From 91

Chapter 2: YOU **CAN** TEACH AN OLD DOG NEW TRICKS 107
    Identify the Negative Habit 109
    Eliminate the Triggers 110
    Create a Positive Counteractive Habit 111
    Develop the Master Habit— GET UP 114
    The *Put In A Dent* Technique 116

Chapter 3: THE POWER OF LITTLE STEPS 123

Part Two: the Practice

Chapter 4: NUTRITION 137
- How *Not* to Diet 139
- The Reason We Gain Weight 152
- Listen To Your Body 159
- Food Additives— Anything But Simple 164
- Genetically Modified Foods 178
- Organic Foods 182
- A Simple Plan 187

Chapter 5: FITNESS 227
- We Are Made To Move 229
- Stretch 236
- Keep It Moving 243
- Take It Outside 245
- Up A Notch— Follow a Workout Routine 246
  - Working Out at Home— 1 Year Fitness Program 251
  - Working Out at the Gym— 1 Year Fitness Program 257
- Hiring A Personal Trainer 272

Afterword 275

We were all given the gift of beginning at birth.

We are also given the gift of a *new* beginning with each day the sun rises— every night we go to bed and, as we take in the first breath of morning air, we are born again.

Then, there is the moment of NOW— now that is truly a new beginning! Forget about *"I'll start on Monday"*, forget about New Year's resolutions— they rarely work. NOW you can make a decision. NOW you can make a life-promoting choice. NOW you can make a change.

If you truly believed in the reality of who you are— the creative, unique individual that God always sees— and let it pierce outwards through your destructive habits like a bullet, then you would have truly figured out yourself. And the ocean of unanswered questions harboring in your mind will instantly vanish, because you figured out the single answer you needed to hear.

Acknowledgements

My sincere gratitude and love to my editor, Vanessa Mileto, for her patience and beyond-her-years professionalism.

I would also like to thank Connie Smith for reading my manuscript and for providing me with valuable insight as well as beautiful words of encouragement.

Last but not least, my deepest love to my daughter Alesa, my husband Giuseppe and, of course, Olaf my rescue cat, for their positive energy and for putting up with my tantrums while going through the labour pains of writing this book.

Introduction

When something in life doesn't go our way the most ridiculous thing to believe is that we know it all. There is always something new to be learned. In order to make definite changes— whether it's getting rid of a simple annoying pattern or beating a deeply ingrained habit such as smoking— you'll need something to always fall back on, rely on, believe, and that is knowledge. What we achieve and don't achieve in life has a lot to do with the amount of knowledge we are willing to allow to go past our ears and make it stay in our brains. It is continuously being receptive to information that opens eyes and minds, nurtures curiosity, helps us expand and grow. Knowledge has the ability to lift us from the lowest point of understanding to unimaginable heights of realization and ideas we never thought we could possibly entertain. It provides us with the tools, which in turn gives us the confidence we need to change for the better.

For as long as I could remember I felt pressed down by one bad habit after another— I know firsthand how destructive the effects of bad habits can be. They never stop at, for example, weight gain in the case of overeating. They seep into other areas of life. My habit of sugar binging, which started when I was a small child and went on until my 30s, used to make me feel unreliable as a person. My habits of overeating and eating unhealthy foods, which led me to experience high physical discomfort and eventually started to translate into weight gain, used to make me feel powerless. My habit of smoking was double as dumb and unhealthy in my case, considering that my livelihood depended on the health of my vocal cords—knowing that, yet not being able to overcome it, used to make me feel weak and incapable as a person. My habit of being extremely self-judgmental and thinking very little of myself pushed me to constantly reach for an unrealistic perfection in order to make up for my "lacks"; it gave me a painful low self-esteem and deeply affected the way I was presenting myself in front of other people. Subsequently, it was one of the reasons I attracted individuals who suppressed me to unimaginable levels. And last, but definitely not least, my habit of negative internalizing (one I consider the most devious of all) led me to feel constantly downhearted; something which caused me severe anxiety and over the years morphed into panic attacks.

For decades, all of the above translated into obstacles firmly cemented between my goals and me. Although I never experienced serious addictions, my damaging behaviors were enough to deeply affect me on all levels. Even though I never ceased working hard on improving my craft, my poor habits stopped me from experience life to its fullest and becoming the best version of myself.

Looking back though, I realized all that happened because of one thing alone: I didn't have the right piece of information. No amount of hope, positive affirmations, or even hard work, was going to be enough to get my butt to where I wanted, unless I added into the mix the information, the knowledge, of what was physically taking place inside my head— unless I understood that it all starts in the brain. Regardless of how weak you feel in front of a particular habit, having the right data gives you the confidence and support to decide differently in what can be a very difficult time. When you don't feel in charge— which is mainly how one feels when enslaved by unwanted habits— it's mostly because of lack of a particular piece of information. Because if you knew exactly what happens physiologically in your brain at the time of birth of a habit, you would definitely and utterly think twice before engaging in it. You would stop perpetuating a negative behavior long before it latches onto your brain, turns into a habit or an addiction, and takes control of your life.

Knowledge makes you stronger; it is the safety net stretching quietly under the acrobatics of life— once acquired, it will always be there, ready to catch you in the eventuality you jump too high and miss the bar.

For years I searched for an answer and finally stumbled over some concepts that made the most sense to me. Something I'm personally very grateful for is the specialists, doctors, researchers, teachers out there, people who are making consistent efforts to put out the right kind of information and help keep the truth in light; people who truly care for others as well as this beautiful, tolerant planet we're living on. It's because of these wonderful people that I also had the opportunity to learn. As I continuously studied their work in various areas, then put my own spin of simplicity on it, I finally started seeing consistent results. And this is what I'm going to relay here: the knowledge I was so incredibly lucky to have come across over the years, which saved me from my own bunch of negative habits.

On another note, *HABITS RULE YOU* does not address severe conditions such as alcohol and drug addictions. Even though at their core they are still habits, these addictions cannot be fully overcome by reading a book. Rather, they have to be taken care of with the help of a qualified practitioner, and in some cases in a specialized facility. However, I do hope this book will offer supporting information, enough to strengthen the desire to get better and help one remember of the powerful resources that undeniably exist within.

You'll notice throughout the book that I mention various professionals and programs. These are meant to be recommendations only and because they have been working wonderfully for me, I made a decision to share them with you as well. If health conditions are present, I strongly recommend that you do not make any changes in your diet or fitness, unless you first consult with your health care provider.

Now a bit of background on myself.

I grew up in Romania, in a beautiful town nestled by the Blue Danube River called Galati. At 6 years old I discovered music and singing which, as years went by, became a truly meditative escape for me. Living under the restrains of the communist regime, we didn't have much; but my parents did everything they could to make my being on stage possible. It was because of their unconditional support that I was able to pursue my passion full time— went on to study Music Theatre at the university in Bucharest and performed in beautiful theatres across the country.

In my mid twenties I moved to Canada with my now ex-husband. Although it was heartbreaking to leave behind everything I'd ever known, in reality it was a blessing to be living in what I regard as one of the best countries in the world. Unfortunately, within a few years I plunged on a downward spiral and lost everything I'd built since I was a child. I ended up in a Toronto hospital weighted down by severe anxiety, heart palpitations and a plethora of other health issues, on the brink of divorce— to say that I was feeling lost and confused would be an understatement.

After a while of hanging out in the victim zone, I finally came to the liberating conclusion that throwing my life to waste was not something I was willing to settle for. So I picked myself up and proceeded to start all over.

Somehow...

I wanted to resume my singing but the education and experience I had weren't exactly prerequisites for any of the jobs listed in the classified section of the Toronto newspapers. However, bills needed to be paid so I had no choice but to reconsider what to do for a living. At least temporarily.

After a couple of years of working in telemarketing and door-to-door sales, I thought it would be a good idea to look for a more gratifying type of occupation— and that was the blessed time when I learned of a concept totally new to me called *continuing education*. Next, I went to Seneca College in Toronto and picked up one of their course catalogues. While reading over the areas of study, I stumbled upon the Fitness Leadership program and the proverbial bulb lit up in my overwhelmed brain— getting an education in Fitness seemed like a pretty good idea to play with until I got my music career back on track.

Or so I thought…

It was during the very first day of school that I had the surprise of my life; I discovered that deep inside I had a genuine passion for wellness. Learning about how quickly and positively the remarkable human body responds when treated with respect then having the opportunity to share this knowledge with other people looking for answers, were the reasons why I ended up working in the fitness field for more than a decade.

On another note, you'll notice that I bring God into the equation quite often, so let me give you a bit of information on where I come from spiritually.

I was born and raised as an Orthodox, a Christian religion similar to Catholicism. I always feel at home in any Orthodox church, anytime, anywhere in the world. As a matter of fact, back in Romania when I used to go on tour singing, the first thing I would do once I arrived in the next city was find the closest church and have a quiet hour. Then I would get back to the hotel and get ready for my show. However, although I was born in this religion, I prefer to call myself a *spiritual Christian*. I believe in Jesus— He is my role model and my guiding light. I believe in a merciful, loving God as the Father of us all, Who gave us free will so that we can choose wisely (hopefully) and decide the curves and turns in the path He's entrusted each of us with. I believe He wants the best for all of us and that He is always present. I believe knowing where we originate from is imperative, as the impression we have of ourselves shows through everything that we do— if we believe we're unworthy, we project a certain level of negativity. But if we understand we're God's children and truly feel that, we become a reflection of His love.

When I mention *spirituality*, I don't mean it from a standpoint of a certain religion, belief, sect, or anything close to that. Being spiritual is being in touch with our soul— that part of us invisible to the physical eye, and which we're yet to understand the vastness of. *Soul* is the essence of who we really are: a brightest light belonging entirely to God. A light that can never be tarnished and which goes on forever. It is what gives us inspiration (in-spirit) and is the source of our intuition. Once we make a habit of tapping into the vast knowledge of our soul and make our every day decisions from that standpoint rather than our egos, we can only become more compassionate; we shift from having a perception to having no perception at all and as a result, we are free of judgment.

I believe we all can— and maybe should— strive to achieve that, regardless of whether we call ourselves Spiritual, Christian, Buddhist, or whatever label we may decide to take on.

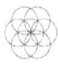

I would like to also clarify a word that's being used in many different contexts and under various meanings, and which I'm bringing in as well: *ego*. What is this *ego*?

Some say (and I happen to have the same opinion) that ego comes from an exaggerated sense of self-importance— wanting to be right, needing to impress, having arrogance, anger, lack of kindness or compassion; that we each create an ego for ourselves, which becomes more defined and in charge the more we dwell on these negative aspects.

Others think of ego as the "enemy"— this gives the ego its own identity and a clearly defined purpose: to create discord and dysfunction.

There are quite a few different perspectives on what the ego is, but I think the point here is not necessarily to find the perfect definition. Whether people create the ego or it originates from somewhere else entirely, I choose to look at it through a simpler perspective. Despite all the negative connotations we give the ego, I believe it exists for a very clear purpose: to give meaning to our free will. Free will would not be of much use to us if what we had to choose from were only positive. It is when we have to decide between what we define as "good" and "bad" that we fully exercise this God-given gift. And it is when we consistently make positive choices (which over time turn into our good habits) that we come into our own and grow. Ego gives us a platform to make that possible.

When it comes to nutrition and fitness in particular, there could be a combination of changes or adjustments you might have to try in order to achieve your desired success. Altering the diet alone might work wonders for some, while only partial for others. It is possible that aside from a diet change you might also have to make adjustments in your fitness habits— sprinting doesn't always work for everybody; while it can work great for some, others might get better results from doing boxing or

Tai Chi. When it comes to the physical body, although our systems work similarly, we're different in the way we react to certain foods and exercise routines. The good news is that your intelligent body will never fail in letting you know right away if what you just ate, or the workout you just completed, is going to have a positive impact or not so much.

One other thing you'll notice throughout the book is that I repeat certain points. Repetition is of utter importance when it comes to creating or discreating habits, as it creates a better understanding. And fully understanding something— which hardly ever comes from reading it once— is one of the most important factors when it comes to creating and sustaining positive habits (or *life-promoting* as I like to call them).

The book is divided in 2 parts. Part 1 (the Theory), gives an in-depth view on the anatomy of habit; how habits form and what makes them have so much pull over one's behavior. It covers the 5 important aspects I believe are important to be taken into consideration before one starts eliminating harmful habitual behaviors and/or creating positive ones. In Part 2 (the Practice), you'll find practical applications in Nutrition and Fitness.

I would recommend that you don't skip Part 1, looking for a quick fix in Part 2. The first half gives important information on how to eliminate harmful habits, how to create new positive ones, and most importantly, how to keep them long-term. Although the focus of this book is how one can improve in the areas of nutrition and fitness, the tips and information I put together in Part 1 can be easily applied to creating positive habits and discreating negative ones in all areas of life. Whether you're interested in improving your diet, fitness level, thought pattern or emotions, all habits are created based on the same formula.

Lastly, the combination of ideas and theories I present in this book is what I guide myself by. It is what helped me overcome my own bunch of negative habitual behaviors— from a long-term sugar addiction, eating unhealthy foods and overeating, to smoking, chronic anxiety, procrastination, negative internalizing, striving for perfection and being judgmental toward myself. It is what gives me the confidence to keep going forward toward what I know in my heart I'm capable of achieving, while weeding out the negative comments and unsupportive opinions coming from the "peanut gallery"— regardless of whether they are family members, friends, or people holding regarded positions in our society.

In a nutshell, my philosophy is this: *never give up*. Never succumb to a situation, a person, a negative habit, or anything else that suffocates your potential. If something bothers you, instead of making it your life sentence, go on a quest to finding the answer. Something I learned over the years is that once a problem is born, the answer is born along with it— we just have to *want* to find it.

The beauty of it is that in most cases the answer is not at all complicated, and it can be found in the simplicity of life.

Why Nutrition and Fitness?

I decided to tackle these topics in particular as they are areas in which I personally experienced great extremes, and because of the extensive research I did in my pursuit to finding answers I gathered ample information. Let me touch on these two areas one by one.

Nutrition

When I was growing up in Romania, there were no "conventionally grown", "organically grown", or "traditionally grown" vegetables— we simply had *vegetables*. We didn't need to put farming in different categories because all foods were grown the same: the way our ancestors did. (Unfortunately, that's not entirely the case anymore.)

When I moved to North America, within weeks I started feeling as if a train hit me. I began having headaches, skin rashes, acne (which looked more like volcano eruptions on my face and neck), eczema on my knees and elbows, an unusual pain going down my spine, irritability, increased anxiety, panic attacks, heart palpitations, irritable bowel syndrome, plus a general feeling of "I'm not here" (which I learned later is *brain fog*). Constipation— a totally new concept to me— seemed to be at home in my body, to the point where I became genuinely jealous of people suffering from diarrhea!

The interesting part is that every time I traveled back to Europe the troubling symptoms disappeared; as soon as I returned to North America, within days I felt sick again.

In a desperate attempt to find an answer, I repeatedly went to see my family doctor. But just as repeatedly, she told me there was nothing wrong with me— which was very puzzling to me considering the way I was feeling. After a few years of basically begging her to fix me and her coming back with "Everything is within normal range", she eventually recommended that I saw a psychotherapist.

Between us, I most likely needed one— but not for my constipation, that's for sure!

About 4 years later I made the decision to go to college and study Fitness Leadership, a program where I learned about fitness, nutrition, sports injuries, anatomy and physiology, among other topics. Studying these subjects gave me the knowledge I needed to finally get my "AHA" moment: it was the drastic change in my diet that came with moving to a new continent that was making me sick. My system— which up until then was accustomed to very simple foods— was all of a sudden inundated with strange things like monosodium glutamate (MSG), food coloring, high fructose corn syrup, pesticides, modified corn starch, artificial sweeteners... As soon as I started making healthier food choices (which eventually turned into my long-term eating habits), my bothersome symptoms disappeared one by one. (And yes, I changed my family doctor!)

However, the valuable information I learned from textbooks became even more precious and potent the moment I remembered and took into consideration the wisdom and simplicity of my own roots. It was this *combination* of information that brought me to a simple yet effective conclusion, which has been working wonderfully for my family and I for the past 18 years and which is what I'm going to relay to you in the following chapters.

Fitness

For as long as I could remember, I had low self-esteem due to what I perceived as having a "not perfectly proportioned" body. I always hid my very tiny shoulders under sleeves with enormous shoulder pads, regardless of season. My drawers were filled with shoulder pads of various shapes and colors, each one topped with a safety pin, ready to be used anytime on any garment I wanted.

Once I began studying fitness, I learned that the body can— to a certain degree— be reshaped. I was so amazed by the results I achieved after only 4 months of training, that I actually had the gall to go into fitness modeling competitions.

One day I was working in a fitness facility carrying out my preliminary fitness assessment on a young woman, when I had an astonishing surprise. I asked her my usual question, "What is your fitness goal?", and her reply was "I want to have shoulders like you." Immediately a question exploded in my mind: "She wants to have shoulders like

WHO?!" If, during the time when shoulder pads were my absolute most important fashion accessory, someone would have told me that in only a few years my very tiny shoulders were going to be a fitness goal for other women, I would've honestly, unequivocally been convinced they were making fun of me.

It's easy to assume at this point that achieving better looking shoulders was my main fitness goal, since I was so self-conscious of them. And it probably would've been, had I not been dealing with something far more important at the time: my health. It was the health issues I was dealing with that drove me into the gym. Improving my physical appearance was only the byproduct of my working out due to the desire to be healthy and feel better.

I will talk in a later chapter about how any reason that motivates you into loosing weight will work, no matter what that reason might be. As long as it keeps you on the right track. There is nothing wrong with wanting to lose weight to make a good impression at your 20-year high school reunion. But what about *after* the party? What about after the vacation, what about after the wedding? In order to be successful in the long run, you will need something that doesn't just motivate you but inspire you.

Remarkable, but most importantly *lasting* results take place when you get your reasons right. Decide to be physically more active while keeping health as your main goal, and you'll be surprised at how easy it is to choose right over wrong and also be patient in the process. This will ultimately translate into healthier habits: you will work *with* your body rather than against it, you will not abuse it with extreme diets and dreadful fitness routines. In return, your body will quickly show you its true adaptability and regenerative capability.

Habits –Good *and* Bad– Rule Us

I could sum up this entire book in one short sentence: MAKE LIFE-PROMOTING CHOICES CONSISTENTLY. That means that whenever you are faced with having to make a choice, you decide to do the right thing. No matter how many lousy excuses your automatic pilot comes up with, no matter how many lies such as "I can't", "It's hard", "It's impossible", "Not realistic", "Against all odds", "It's not what *they* expect of me", "I'm too old" surface on your mind, you choose to make a life-promoting choice. Why is this important? Because every habit starts with a choice. What do you call the first time you put a cigarette in your mouth? You call it a "choice"— you chose to do so. Once you make that choice and continue making it, you facilitate the birth of a habit. How strong your smoking habit may become is another story, as it depends upon how long you choose to light up that cigarette.

Make life-promoting choices consistently— there. If you got that, then I'm telling you right now you can put the book down 'cause you don't need to read the rest of it.

However, if you're like me, welcome to the club! You're most definitely not alone. The truth is that my story is not one of those we often watch in an inspiring film highlighting the difficult life of a woman who one night has an inspiring dream, then she gets up in the morning and makes a choice that positively and permanently changes the rest of her life. No, that's not what happened with me, not even close. I'm one of those stubborn-for-no-apparent-reason individuals who needed to experience heartache over the course of many years, before I finally realized that I'm not a soccer ball available to be kicked around by some frikin' lousy habits I created by default. I'm a person who, after receiving a wakeup call pretty loud and clear, made a choice to change but shortly after she fell back into her old ways. Then she was lucky enough to get another loud and clear sign, made the choice, and fell back again.

Then again…

And again…

For a long time I expected my life to miraculously change just because I woke up in the morning with a new choice in my head. If you, too, expect that, think again. No doubt, making the choice is what ignites the change.

But how do you sustain it?

There is something powerful working on your behalf; something which won't give up its power over you unless you take it seriously: your habits. Habits are the driver behind everything that we do and everything we don't do. It may seem like habits work in mysterious ways but the truth is, we create them that way in the first place—

we tend to get sloppy and let our default mechanisms take over, resulting in bad habits that work against our goals and dreams. Then we identify ourselves with them and let them govern our life.

Now, doesn't that sound crazy when you really think about it?!

After more than 20 years of experiencing unwanted incidences in one department or another, I finally came to the liberating conclusion that nothing happened *to* me. Some of the things I experienced would not have been in my life (or at least their intensity would've been much less) had I not told them "Come on in".

But why is it that we say "Yes" to pain? Why is it that we accept— some of us even seem to love— drama?

We each have different reasons to do so, but mostly it is because of the habits ruling us in the background— habits we've been unknowingly practicing and reinforcing for years. Although we don't always realize, even negative habits are achieved by repetition. Yes, it takes consistent practice to get to the point of going straight to the couch after eating dinner. Over and over again we hear it's best to have a walk after dinner, but not many seem to be able to do that. Some of us try but too soon give up, simply because the habit deeply ingrained in the brain won't allow the change. But you may not be aware of what is actually happening. You may think you're lazy or ignorant toward your own health. You look at others as they do the "right thing" and maybe envy them for it… The good news is that although the autopilot is firmly set in its seat, your clarity of goal, your persistence and patience, can undeniably push it off the driver seat.

All of us— without exception— have the potential of finding meaning in life regardless of the conditions we were born under, regardless of where we are at any point in our life. We all have an equal opportunity to choose between acquiring bad habits and zigzagging with our God-given purpose or creating positive habits and steering straight toward it. There is always something we can do because we possess a *mind* and *free will*. When we understand the power of our mind and the tremendous gift of free will we were given— then add a little bit of patience in the mix— each of us is capable of achieving our own definition of success. But we have to recognize and shake off the habits that have been holding us back and replace them with habits which, put simply, promote *life*.

"We are creatures of habits"— isn't that something we repetitively say? It's those habits we so lightly acknowledge that shape experiences, even characters. Do you have a habit of drinking excessively or occasionally? Do you have a habit of wanting to learn or do you have an "I know it all" habit? Do you have a habit of being physically active consistently, or do you have a habit of making fitness your New Year's resolution and drop it by the time March comes along? Do you have a habit of making excuses or taking responsibility? Do you have— what is probably the most deceiving of all— the habit of negative internalizing? Yes we are what we eat, and yes we are what we think. But in the end, it all narrows down to one thing: we are our habits. Because the kind of foods we eat on a regular basis is a habit; how we take our coffee is a habit; the state of mind we're in most of the time is a habit, therefore, our overall emotions become a habit; our usual reaction to people cutting us off on the road is a habit.

Unfortunately, most of the times we start paying attention to our negative habits when the pain or some other form of negative result becomes imminent and pushes over the edge. Let's dissect one of today's most notorious habits: watching TV. And by that, I mean in excess. (In case you're wondering, watching superhero and princess movies back to back in your pajamas on the occasional Saturday doesn't fall in this category. ...At least I hope it doesn't or else I'm in big trouble!) For the sake of the argument though, let's assume you watch TV excessively. If your doctor said you had a terminal illness which can be completely cured by not watching TV for one year, would you do it? Of course you would! You would decisively, unequivocally do it. It wouldn't be easy in the beginning, but the new belief you just acquired— that you will be healed by not watching TV— will trigger a firm decision to take place in your mind. No questions asked, you will bypass your automatic pilot and consciously make the change.

But do we really need a strong wakeup call before we get up and do something despite our bad habits chaining us down? Do we really need someone telling us that we are going to die, in order to realize we do have a will?

And how about that treasured, sometimes secret desire— how about your DREAM? What is the habit you created that muffled your enthusiasm and chained down your desire to achieve it? Failing to recognize the reality of who we are by not following our dreams is a disastrous habit entertained too often. And we take it far too lightly. We find all the excuses in the world why we won't go for it, yet another horrible habit too many of us easily fall pray to.

What if God came to you and said that by following your dream you will discover a kind of peace you can't even conceive yet? What if God told you that your dream is who you are— *your dream is you*— and not believing that it can happen is the same as not trusting in Him? What if God told you all that? Would you get up, grab your bad habit by its feet, spin it forcefully around in circles above your head, then quickly let go of it with the knowing that it will never come back because *you said so*?

Would you do that?

You may think, "What are the odds of God coming to *me* to say all that?" Well, He does. Close your eyes and imagine you are living as who you always wanted to be. You see yourself in that very position, sure of yourself, peaceful, and secure. That indescribable feeling is God telling you all of the above and infinitely more. It is God telling you that you are completely able because He gave you the ability— this is the real you, wake up already, make the decision and stick with it.

You will notice throughout this book that most of the examples I give are personal. The reason for this is to give you the confidence that everything I say is very much possible, because it was possible for me. You might find some of my life details intense, maybe even slightly depressing at times, but that's not without reason. Being pushed to my limit forced me into discovering the true resilience of the human spirit and ultimately showed me who I truly was. I realized that I was absurdly much stronger than I thought. I understood the massive importance of "waking up", dare to assess myself— my mind— and clarify *exactly* what *I* wanted. Not what I was dictated to want by others who were themselves disconnected from the truth.

I soon learned that what I truly wanted was to be genuinely hopeful, to develop, to freely express myself through my passion and the things I love— which, in fact, is something I always had the freedom to choose.

However, I didn't write this book to be a crybaby and tell you of my past troubles. I wrote this book to tell you that after all the baloney I put myself through— yes, it was *me* who accepted it in the first place— I finally came to this liberating conclusion: WE DO NOT HAVE TO FALL IN ORDER TO LEARN.

Making perfect choices every day for the rest of our lives is not possible. I get it. But going to the other extreme and tolerating the "rock bottom" theory as a requirement to learn or wake up, is downright wrong in my opinion. It is a form of justification to cover up past errors by telling oneself, "There was a reason for that, I learned something, eh..." I used to believe that, until one day when I realized that what I really "learned" is that I delayed myself from reaching my destiny. I learned that I did not take advantage of the creative power I was given and which I was supposed to use for my own good and others'. I learned that I kept this whole world a little bit behind because of my lack of genuine interest in who I was.

We keep letting our crippling judgment conclude on our behalf that carrying a cross is inevitable, even necessary. What if instead, we put our proverbial cross down and solely identified our life with the miracle of Resurrection? I hate to break it to some, but Jesus underwent the crucifixion so we don't have to. *"Do not make the pathetic error of clinging to the old rugged cross."* He says in *A Course in Miracles*. *"The only message of the crucifixion is that you can overcome the cross. Until then you are free to crucify yourself as often as you chose."*

So no, you do not need a wakeup call in order to learn, in order to be wiser or more aware. You don't have to let yourself experience painful lows or go through agony and despair in order to succeed. You don't need to have a *story* in order to make it on the front page of your local newspaper. You can make it so that you build your awareness and lift yourself *before* you let your cheeks crash on the cold cement floor, before you possibly throw years of your life to waste. People used to ask me "How did you take all the abuse from that person?", or "I don't understand, you're working so hard, why is it that you're still struggling...?" You know what my answer used to be? "You need a good story to be on the Oprah show". People thought I was kidding but the truth is, I wasn't. Not that I was consciously choosing to have negative experiences, but I used to believe that paying my dues by tolerating useless hardships was necessary in order to learn and (hopefully) succeed. Yes, you read that right, "hopefully" succeed— falling rock bottom never gives immunity against an unsuccessful life.

Falling rock bottom is unnecessary. Nowhere does it say that being a victim or that paying your dues by suffering is required in order to eventually thrive. And if anybody tells you that, turn your back at them and run as fast as you can. You don't need monuments to be erected in your memory as a constant reminder of your sacrifices. You want to live NOW and live well. You want to live successful, strong, creative, proud of who you are. The only monument you want— if you really must have one, ha ha— is one honoring you as an inspirer, honoring you as a bringer of light and hope, honoring you as an example of living with purpose.

So how do we achieve that? How do we get to where we want (not necessarily free of stress and aggravation because that's not realistic on this planet) but possibly with less stress and aggravation? How do we create a better, purposeful life?

How do we get more of what we really want?

I say we do that by paying close attention to our every day habits. As Aristotle said, "*We are what we repeatedly do. Excellence, then, is not an act, but a habit.*"

Did you ever think that behind all your "ups" and "downs" there might be certain habits you created at some point in your past? Did you ever wonder which habits are laying behind that bothersome issue that keeps you from falling asleep at night? Did you ever wonder what habits are responsible for your shortcomings or that unfulfilled dream?

On the other hand, did you ever wonder which habits are laying behind the positive outcomes in your life, behind your successes and victories? Being aware of the positive habits behind your achievements is just as important as being aware of your hindering habits.

Do you know which habits rule you?

Give Simplicity A Chance

We're living in an extraordinary time, with technology advancing at incredible speed— it truly is remarkable how far we've come in the last 10 years alone.

On the other hand, there is a side effect to putting on horse visors and racing towards technological perfection: we tend to forget about the concept of *simplicity*. All this speeding forward leaves behind a trail of pollution that chokes and blinds us, quite literally in some cases. Sometimes it gets so strong, we lose our common sense; we reach out, hoping to grab onto something that can give us a sense of direction and stability. Sometimes we get lucky and out of the smoky air we catch the right advice. Unfortunately, more often than not, what we catch and hold on to with all our hope is something that gives a false, temporary sense of support. As a result, our minds become more and more complex and twisted, making it increasingly harder to grasp the concept of simplicity.

Far too easily we get caught up in trying to understand the non-understandable. But the non-understandable is exactly that: *non-understandable*. So why would you even begin to waste your time attempting to get it? No matter how much effort you put into trying to comprehend which bread is best to eat; which yogurt has the most acidophilus; if you should eat whole eggs or egg whites only; how many hours is optimal to sleep at night; which mattress lullabies you to sleep faster; what heavily advertised workout machine or programs printed on DVDs or new pills are best for quick weight loss; if it's better to work out at home or is hiring a pricey personal trainer the answer; whether to use spf 20 or 30 or 50; which hair care products give the smoothest hair; whether to drink tap water or spend money on bottled water— which raises yet another daunting question "Which brand is healthier?"; ...you will most likely not get a straight answer because it's all too complicated.

The only consistent point in all these fads is "RESULTS MAY VARY".

For every one of the areas I mentioned above there is a multitude of "answers" ready to catch your attention and your hard-earned money. *"I don't know what's good anymore."* — that becomes the main concern applying to almost everything, from diets to fitness programs to even religious beliefs. Allowing ourselves to get overwhelmed and off balance by the countless processed foods, the extreme weight loss promising diets and everything else in between, is playing hide-n-seek with our wellbeing. And it's complicating our lives. You will not get your answer if you keep looking there because what you're looking to find relief in is, in many cases, an illusion created by expensive marketing campaigns.

Someone suggested that I wrote 2 books on the subjects of Nutrition and Fitness, instead of covering them in one book. For about a second I considered it, but then I quickly realized that it would've gone against my message of simplicity— and God knows we need simplicity in our lives more than ever. As my fellow ladies would understand, we barely find the time to put 15 minutes aside to take a relaxing bath once in a while, let alone read a 300-page book on the topic of shakes alone. The reason why so many of us struggle with issues such as weight gain and chronic stress (to name just a few) is because we foolishly fell into the habit of disregarding the concept of simplicity.

I don't mean to minimize the complexities of life. We live in an extraordinary time; a time that is overflowing with precious new discoveries. On the other hand, it is this ever-increasing mass of information that makes pinpointing the right answer harder and harder. For the longest time I was incredibly confused by the vastness of information available and followed whatever screamed the loudest. In the end, I didn't get long-lasting results— wasted my money at the very best and got hurt at the very worst. So the question is, how do we recognize what's real out of the avalanche of information spinning around in circles above our (sometimes) fogged brains? I say we can pinpoint it by looking for the simplicity in it— if it gets complicated, it's not it. It has to be simple. How will you know what's simple? You'll know because you will understand it. You'll know because it's easy to follow. You'll know because once you hear it, you will not be overwhelmed with questions.

Today, more than ever, we need to hold on to the simplicity of our roots. Then, when combined with the right new piece of information, we can arrive at the best possible answer. An answer that has the capacity to inspire others to be open to it; an answer which will not ask compromise of anybody or anything (including our resilient planet).

The good news is that no matter how far off we've gone simplicity is never too far away. Simplicity is what we started with; it is in our roots, ingrained in our DNA. At any point in time we can simply decide to rely on it, should we choose to dismiss what confuses us. As soon as we give simplicity a fair chance, we will not only understand what we need to understand, but truly know— simply because it's already in us.

During the time that I worked in the fitness industry I've assisted many people, each with their own unique concerns and fitness goals. My role in my clients' success never stopped with the last paid session. How they were keeping up after, on their own, was also important to me. Years later, I was more than surprised to learn that it wasn't the structured fitness routines I put them on that stayed with them the most, but a minimal piece of advice: "Keep it simple". I didn't learn about that in school or anywhere in particular but somehow, I felt it was the most direct path to wellbeing. Keeping it simple took me on no detours because simplicity is, and always will be, predictable.

Unfortunately, simplicity is not always taken as a valid answer. And I don't mean this only in the areas of nutrition and fitness, but in general. Disregarding its validity became such a habit, that as soon as we hear something is simple, we become instantaneously judgmental, critical, even resentful.

A few years ago, I heard of a child who was revered by many around the globe for his spiritual teachings. He was giving speeches, raising awareness in people, doing his part with the intention of creating a better world. I learned about this child while driving one day, when the radio announcer mentioned that the night before he had given a presentation at a large venue in Toronto. One of the announcers played a short recording of the child's speech. In this excerpt, the child was asked by an audience member, if he were to give one piece of advice, what would it be? With what I could perceive was a smile on his face, the child answered, "*Be happy— that is the answer to life*".

The radio hosts chuckled slightly sarcastically at the simplicity of the child's answer. When I heard them somewhat turning this boy's answer into a joke, I felt there was something very off here. How could these people— whose job supposedly is to make their listeners' day better— put this concept down, disrespect it with such ease? What if THIS IS IT? What if this is *the* answer? What if the toughest pain, the biggest disappointment, the most severe anxiety... what if everything we battle in life can be resolved by a simple answer such as BE HAPPY?

Why do we disregard simplicity so easily?

This might seem like I'm departing from the topic of the book, but I strongly believe having constructive habits in nutrition and fitness is not achieved by focusing solely on nutrition and fitness. The same fitness routine or eating habits will give one kind of results to a person who makes an effort to consistently have general hopeful thoughts, and will give different results to a person who has a general negative outlook towards life. We are extremely complex beings, with our brains being at the top of the list— the brain is where it's at. What goes on in there is the initiator and the driver; it is the reason and the answer to all that we do and don't do, to what we achieve and don't achieve. Thus, it's important to have a sincere, unbiased look at everything that's going on in there.

What we need most right now is simplicity, and I mean in all areas of our life. However, what we eat is particularly a major concern that too many of us have. We gain more weight than ever, easier than ever. You probably heard the statistics by now. Steve Bradt, Harvard staff writer notes: *"Researchers at Harvard University say America's obesity epidemic won't plateau until at least 42 percent of adults are obese."* I believe this is happening because we forgot to think simple. And we had a good reason to do so, considering the complicated information being put out almost by the day. We almost had no choice but to forget simplicity. And that's all right. But now it's time we claim it back.

Firstly, we have to shake our minds off all pretenses; unless we do so, we cannot comprehend the magnificence of simplicity because simplicity is difficult to be understood by an already invested mind. You want to clear your mind of everything that makes you wonder over and over again and consistently gives you a relief-less answer. Simplicity cannot coexist alongside the ever confusing "How many calories should I eat in a day?" I know that works for some. However, if you're like me, if counting every single bite that goes in your mouth doesn't appeal to you, then you might want to give this concept a try.

I can't guarantee that by applying simplicity in your life all your problems will be solved, that would be silly. But I thought since "Results may vary" is something we've settled on for a while now, we might as well make our life easier by creating a habit of making simpler choices. Doing that gave me the least stress while trying to accomplish something. The only pressure I can foresee is in the beginning, when unlearning the complicated information that hasn't been working for you. Depending on how old those habits are, it will take a certain amount of time to eliminate them. Nevertheless, if you stick to your plan, eventually the situation will go in reverse. Once you grasp the concept of simplicity, it will become easier and easier to decipher between the multitude of choices thrown at you every day. Before you know it, your automatic pilot will be assisting you in making life-promoting choices consistently.

I'll explain later how to keep it simple in each of the areas I decided to tackle in this book. But to give you an idea at this moment, when getting groceries for example. Look for foods that are as close to their original shape and form as possible. Don't even start stressing out trying to figure out which fruit yogurt is best: the one with fruit at the bottom, on top, or anywhere else. Think simple instead: where does yogurt come from? From milk. Milk comes from cows. Does milk originally come filled with fruit blend, juice concentrates, natural flavors, pectin, artificial sweeteners, milk and whey protein concentrates, modified corn starch, modified milk ingredients, locust bean gum, sodium citrate, potassium sorbate or colors? Does it come with its natural fat removed? Of course not. So get the plain, full-fat, the-way-nature-made-it yogurt. Put a teaspoon of jam in a cup (get the most basic one made with real fruit), add plain yogurt on top, and voila! You got a healthier (and more affordable) version of fruit yogurt. EVEN IF YOU DECIDE TO SWITCH TO ORGANIC FOODS, THIS WILL STILL BE MORE AFFORDABLE. (I know, we are terrified of eating full fat. I will explain later how eating full fat *in moderation* is a better choice.)

Keep it simple when you exercise. If you've never exercised before, best is to start simple: take the old-fashioned walk every day, and then pick up the speed as your endurance increases. Don't go searching for the next expensive piece of equipment being marketed with the promise of burning thousands of calories, then lock yourself in your house and barely see the light of day. I'm not saying that those machines don't work, because they do. As a matter of fact, working out on a treadmill indoor is better than not working out at all. But the thing is, that new machine is not going to help you get the results you want unless you get your habits corrected first. There is no device out there that comes with the guarantee that you'll habitually stick to the program. You should ask yourself this question: by always looking for the next fancy machine, or the "right time" to join the gym, or the perfect workout outfits, are you, maybe, trying to find an excuse of some sort? If you were truly willing to make a change, wouldn't you simply put on your old running shoes and get out the door RIGHT NOW?

Many underestimate the importance of walking outside, just because it sounds too simple. Without realizing that aside from increasing blood flow and oxygen supply to the brain, the "simple" walk outside offers remarkable benefits like natural light, sun, and fresh air. We fail to realize the importance of simply breathing in fresh air or letting the warmth of the sun (outside the peak times) touch our skin. We fail to realize the massive importance of being in touch with the outside; that we are part of nature just as much as a tree is part of nature. Put a tree inside the house along with a cell phone glued to its hip, surrounded by computers, Wi-Fi, smart meters, recycled air, forced air heating, air conditioning, possibly even mold, and I'm pretty sure the wellbeing of that tree would be significantly impaired.

Heck, I feel impaired just by talking about it!

We ignorantly removed ourselves from the simplicity and wisdom of the loop of nature. We keep depleting this beautiful planet of its resources and don't always give back. We pulled ourselves out of the natural loop, placed ourselves higher than nature, thinking that we're so smart... And if, hypothetically, there would be a natural disaster and everything we own was destroyed, most of us would have no idea how to even start a fire to cook a meal, let alone survive. At that point our beautiful, sometimes oversized roofs we work so hard to put over our heads would not mean much without their dependency for heat or electricity. Any animal out there— be a squirrel, a mouse, or an elephant— would continue living as if nothing happened. So who is TRULY smarter?

Let's try and give simplicity a chance. My feeling is you won't be disappointed.

Part One: the Theory

Chapter 1

HOW LONG DOES IT TAKE TO FORM A HABIT?

A few years ago, my sister-in-law asked if I could lift one eyebrow. "All women in our family can *do the eyebrow*" she proudly said to me. "Yes I can lift one eyebrow" I responded, and proceeded to lift my left eyebrow without flinching the other one— which impressed her indeed.

That seemingly insignificant episode sparked a question in my mind: why can't I lift my *other* eyebrow? I've been able to lift my left eyebrow for as long as I could remember, but I never gave the other one a thought. If you really think about it, when we contract a muscle group on a regular basis, that particular muscle group gets toned and lifted. Same principle applies to the facial muscles connected to the eyebrows. Logically, if I never lifted my right eyebrow, the muscles involved in moving it are not as used. So wouldn't there be a big chance that over time the right side of my face would be less toned, maybe even droopy?

When my husband, Giuseppe, and I got home that night, I could not get my mind off the eyebrow episode. With a great deal of skepticism that it would even be possible, I went ahead and attempted to lift my "immovable" eyebrow. But just as I expected, it seemed completely dead. I couldn't even begin to feel I had muscles on that side of my face! Every time I was trying to raise my right eyebrow, the left one would lift instead. Then I ran to the mirror and for the first time I noticed my right eyelid was droopy compared to the left one.

I didn't know how to even begin training the right side of my face. The first thought I had was to hold my "active" eyebrow with one hand, while manipulating the other one in an up and down motion with my other hand. As soon as I did that, I got a sensation in the forehead muscles just above my right eyebrow. "So I do have muscles there!" I sarcastically thought to myself. I continued manipulating my right eyebrow with my hand, and *within 5 minutes* I was able to lift it without help.

I was astonished at how easy it was! I still felt a bit strange, as if the upper right side of my face had just got out of a light paralysis or something. Nevertheless, I was doing it. I immediately ran to my husband and shouted with a big smile on my face "This is unbelievable! Five minutes ago I couldn't move my right eyebrow and now I can!!!" Giuseppe looked at me and found it a bit strange; he probably thought, "She lost it— she's finally lost it..." Then he literally patted me on the back and said "That's good... good girl."

That eyebrow episode left a strong impression on me. It was not really about being able to lift an eyebrow. I felt it was about much more than that; something I had a strong feeling could be applied to almost anything. This thought became the seed that led me to start writing a book about habits.

That is a small example of how neuroplasticity works. Neuroplasticity (something I'll be talking about in the next chapter) is the brain's capacity to alter its neural synapses and pathways as a result of changes in behavior. In other words, it is the brain's ability to create new habits. It took me only 5 minutes to create the habit of lifting an eyebrow which I could never move on its own before— it was very easy. All I needed was the awareness that half of my face was beginning to get droopy, plus a bit of patience to put 5 minutes into actually doing it. At the very basics, that is how easy it can be to create *any* habit. Yes, depending on the habit, some will take longer to create and some will take much longer. But the bottom line is that it can be done *once you put your mind to it.* How long it takes doesn't really matter, when you take the outcome into consideration— time passes anyway, so why not make it pass with purpose?

The popular pseudo myth is that a new habit forms between 21 to 28 days. However, research conducted by Phillippa Lally from the *Cancer Research UK Health Behavior Research Centre* points out in the *European Journal of Social Psychologists* that it takes around 66 days of uninterrupted practice before the action has become automatic.

Sixty-six days is a general rule of thumb, but when it comes to beating a bad habit or creating a new one, the exact number of days can't be foreseen. Lally's conclusion was that automaticity can be achieved in as little as 18 days by some, while some might take 254 days and even more. What does that mean? It means that although the number of days cannot be anticipated, the certainty is that if practiced regularly, the habit will eventually become automatic. It means that having patience is of a paramount importance. The body is an extremely intricate machine, with numerous wheels turning continuously day in and day out. Our long-term system of habits created a great momentum, much like a solid set of wheels rolling downhill full force. You cannot possibly bring a speedy wheel to a full stop and instantly make it turn the other way around! You have to be patient— allow your body's wheels to slow down in their due time, then give them a chance to adjust to the new direction and pick up a new momentum. Once they're full speed again, you have your results.

This is when being in control of our habits becomes most feasible— when we don't put a time constraint on our goals and understand that each of us is unique. Therefore, the time it takes each of us to break or create habits is also unique.

Much of what we experience is the result of our every day decisions. Your path might be set at the beginning by God, but you are in charge of walking it— you decide how soon or how late you reach the destiny He pre-envisioned for you. Whatever choices you make via your own free will, in turn creates your every day habits. For example, if you choose to live with the belief that your sugar addiction is beyond your control (as I did for decades), then you will be living a life that *seems* to be directed by this addiction. Yet it is *you* who not only allowed it to happen in the first place but continuously reinforced its power over you. Simply put, you opened the door to it, let it in, and entertained it. Now you have a guest in your mind that's not only rearranging your furniture and taking over your bathroom, but it took the front door key away from you. Now you're stuck outside yourself— which is pretty much how it feels when pushed around by unwanted habits. And this can go pretty far, as the brain is very powerful. When we focus on something long enough the brain not only develops habits, but it can go as far as to create physiological changes in the body in the form of disease, as already showed by scientific researchers. But who directs your brain? You do. And that means you can also create wellness.

But is there a deciding factor in how long it takes each of us to achieve our desired results? What lies behind our ability to create and discreate habits? Why is it that some eliminate a habit of eating excessively within weeks, and others struggle for months before they attain the same result?

Understanding the following 5 concepts was what gave me the background I needed in order to recognize why I was cradling unhealthy behaviors. Once I understood these concepts, I found it much easier to replace my bad habits with constructive ones— from creating a small habit such as having a glass of water with lemon upon waking up in the morning, to eliminating deeply ingrained habits such as smoking and sugar dependency. Understanding or even applying all 5 concepts is not always required in order to succeed. Sometimes one concept alone could be the exact piece of information you needed in order to restore yourself from your own unwanted mind guests.

Here are the concepts:
- The Brain
- The Beliefs
- The Reward
- The Will
- The Knowing

THE BRAIN
— Amygdala and Neural Pathways —

Learning about the physiological changes that happen in the brain when a new habit starts to form as well as during the course of an existing habit is, in my opinion, vital. Reason being, once we know how something works, we also understand its weakness. What makes habits weak? What makes them weak is the fact that the formula to be broken is built within them: exactly how you created them, you also discreate them— by *repetition*. Despite their seeming permanency, habits can be reversed by working your way backwards. I'm not going to claim that that's easy to do. However, regardless of the intensity of your bad habits, once you're committed to using the same formula in reverse, you will become more and more in charge. Making a definite goal then following up with repetition is like following a clear map when you go on a trip; if you stay focused on the right path and have patience, sooner or later *you will reach your destination*.

So what is it that happens physiologically in one's brain when a habit is in its initial stage of formation? The answer lies in:
- The Amygdala
- The Neural Pathways

The Amygdala

Now, what is this amygdala? What is this *rompiballe* (ball breaker) as my Italian husband would say? According to smarter people than I in this area, the amygdala is an almond-shaped limbic system structure, or mass of cells, located within each temporal lobe of the brain. Amygdala is in charge of motivations and emotions, in particular those related to survival— you heard of the fight-or-flight response. The amygdala processes emotions such as fear, anger and pleasure, and it's also responsible for determining what memories are stored and where the memories are stored in the brain. *"Not memories such as your favorite guacamole recipe or where you put your car keys",* Rich Presta explains in his e-book *Your Anxious Brain, "...but memories related to survival."*

Dr. David Perlmutter, International Bestselling Author and empowering neurologist states the following about the amygdala: *"Basically, it is the 'fear center' of the brain, important for our survival as it allows us to respond to dangerous situations reflexively and unconsciously as opposed to actions based upon the deliberate and calculated input from the far more sophisticated prefrontal cortex."*

Our experiences can cause brain circuits to change and form new memories. For example, when witnessing a terrifying event, the amygdala amplifies our perception of what we hear. This heightened perception is frightening, and as a result memories are formed associating the sound with the negative emotion of fright. Then an automatic flight-or-fight response follows. This activity is coordinated by the amygdala, and allows us to respond appropriately to what it perceives as danger. Let's say a child falls off a bicycle and gets hurt. After that experience, just seeing a bicycle may trigger the child's amygdala to take him/her right back to the emotions felt during the incident.

But how does this relate to habits? Since the amygdala is the brain region most associated with our emotional state, scientists say that it plays a crucial role in addiction because of its association with stress, emotions and memory. As a person engages more and more in a certain activity (overeating, sugar binging, etc.), various brain regions associated with their emotional state also increase in activity.

Anything that is a potential danger is recorded by the amygdala, which uses this data to alert if or when a similar situation arises again. In animals, as well as our primitive ancestors, this is a necessary survival tool assessing danger and keeping them safe from being attacked by a wild animal, for example. Today we don't have to worry about that; the "wild animals" setting our amygdalae off are different in our modern-day reality: bills piling up, stressful jobs, deadlines, debts, traffic, busy schedules, having to meet the expectations of others... Although we might refer to them as "life", to the amygdala they are just as real and just as dangerous as being attacked by a wild animal. The amygdala's role is to assist in a life-threatening scenario. Unfortunately, we created a habit of letting this precious little part of our physicality go off whenever it sees fit. Once that happens, a hideous result is created: fear. Now when I say "fear", I don't mean what we might experience when bungee jumping or skydiving. Fear extends into our everyday lives much deeper than sometimes we even begin to recognize; it became a true epidemic that overrules the magnificent innocence of the human spirit. Fear tells you which box you should confine yourself in, putting up an unyielding wall and shutting the door to creativity.

We live in a society where choice based on others' expectations has become commonplace, making fear so deep rooted and so deceiving that it has become part of our existence. We fear that our opinions and decisions may not be good enough. This chronic wanting to be approved of creates more insecurity, more worries, and more anxiety than ever before. Our poor little amygdalae are in a much more difficult position today than our ancestors' used to be. Our stress needle is not going up once in a while anymore, as it used to hundreds of years ago when a mountain lion would show up in the village. The stress needle is now stuck in the "on" position because our modern-day mountain lions attacking us almost every day created a new level of normality, closing in on us like a vicious circle.

However, once you start taking control over your fears, the stress needle will gradually reset itself to the "off" position. Your amygdala will continue doing what it does best, which is make you aware of real dangers. The rest of the time though, it will have to take a step back and comply with what *you* see fit for yourself.

The Neural Pathways

The amygdala however, does not come without its allies, its accomplices if you will: the Neural Pathways. Neurons are made up of nerve cells that transmit nerve signals to and from the brain. These nerve cells, in turn, make up the core of the nervous system, particularly the brain. When you repeatedly do an activity (from learning a new skill or language, to reaching for a specific food, cigarettes, or alcohol for comfort, to being nice to others, nose picking, smiling regularly or not smiling, exercising or not exercising, etc) clusters of neurons work together to create a memory, a new behavior, even a new belief. When neurons connect in this way, they are called *neural pathways*. The reason it's hard to drive a car in the beginning is because there are no neural pathways formed that are conditioned to the specific activity of driving a car. Think of it as actual physical "threads" that start off extremely frail— as you are just introduced to a new behavior— and which turn into thicker and stronger "ropes" as you consistently repeat the behavior. Behind every habit— good and bad— there is always a set of little neural pathways at work. The more you practice, the more robust these neural pathways become, and the stronger your habit; until it reaches the point where it becomes automatic— now it literally acts on your behalf.

As these pathways develop, the collective group of regularly used neural pathways becomes a diagram of how an individual thinks and reacts. A person's character is based on their neural pathway diagrams at each point in time. I always believed that depending on the kind of knowledge a person is willing to be open to, their character can change. But this notion truly solidified in my mind the moment I learned about neural pathways. Accepting new constructive information initiates the birth of new neural pathways, which equals new habits of thought and habits of doing (or not doing) certain things. By simply having better habits, one acts differently, displaying particular character traits.

Through repetition and focused attention, we can forge new neural pathways and thus create new habits. This is what scientists call *neuroplasticity of the brain*. In his book *The Brain that Changes Itself*, Michael Merzenich underlines that practicing a new habit can possibly change billions of new connections between the nerve cells in our neural pathways. Consistent repetition and practice sustained by focused attention are powerful ways to achieve neuroplasticity. Following a disciplined routine (once we are clear as to what result we are seeking) puts neuroplasticity in our total control.

From a practical standpoint, repetition is the key to achieving any goal when it comes to neuroplasticity, thus habit forming. Repetition is the means through which you, I, and everyone else acquired all our habits— both positive and negative. Unless you repeat the task over and over, unless you repeatedly do something, nothing else can get you to the point of developing a habit.

Also, by repeating the act of *not* doing something in spite of your urges, the strong neural pathways in charge of that particular unhealthy habit are going to slowly get weaker and weaker, simply because you're consistently cutting off their fuel. Dr. Perlmutter explains this: "... *So activities need to be maintained if their neural networks are to remain functional. This may sound familiar and distressing, but the 'glass full' aspect of this concept is that it allows for the disappearance of dysfunctional or detrimental networks when attention is directed away from them."*

Imagine this: one day you start walking on a patch of beautiful grass. As you repeatedly walk the same path, the grass slowly gets damaged until it almost disappears, leaving room for a dry pathway that looks very much like a path intended to be there. But if one day you decide to stop walking on it, the grass will slowly come back, until it'll reach the point where the old path is almost completely gone. Same with neural pathways; the more you repeat the behavior, the stronger and more defined the neural pathways. The stronger and more defined the neural pathways, the stronger habit. On the other hand, the more you avoid repeating the unhealthy behavior, the weaker the neural pathway thus the weaker your bad habit.

Poor habits start by sending the signals to the brain followed by focused attention and repetition. Knowing this ahead of time can help one think twice before engaging in any sort of unhealthy behavior. It can make it easier to say "No" to any form of demise, knowing that the second you gave in you initiated the birth of that little "thread" which, should you continue engaging in that particular behavior, is going to eventually put you in a victim position. Knowing this alone, can make it easier to stop a bad habit from forming right then and there.

Allow me to repeat myself: REPETITION IS THE KEY. There is no way around it. There is no magic pill that can help you achieve healthier habits overnight. Repetition is what facilitates the brain to make room for new neural pathways; it's the only way a new habit will literally become physically ingrained in the brain. In the same way, repetition is the key to getting rid of existing bad habits— just like it took time and consistent practice to create them, it will take time and consistent practice to reverse them.

I had a rather unique experience with the process of repetition, at a very young age. Although I didn't know what I was doing at the time, years later I realized what actually took place in my brain...

As a child, composure and quietness were character traits some used when referring to me. However, inside my head there was an engine running steadily. The only time my mind took a rest was when it was drifting away in sleep. The rest of the time it was in a relentless search of things to do.

It was during one of our communist, soul-crushing ballet classes at the age of 10 that I discovered something remarkable. I was not a very skilled dancer, but I was one of the kids who remembered the moves the fastest. Because of this, I and a couple of other girls were occasionally granted short breaks. But the privilege of taking a break didn't come without a stone hard condition: we had to sit on the floor with our legs crossed and not move or talk— in other words, do NOTHING. This was agony to me! As the teacher was counting the beats and screaming at the other girls, an idea came to mind: to count the letters in his sentences. "Liliana, turn left you stupid!", the ballet instructor would scream. In my head I would section his words, place them in equal groups, then come up with the number of letters: 24. "The other left Liliana" the teacher would shout. "19 letters" I would quietly say to myself. My impatience soon reduced by the intensity of this new activity— I enjoyed doing it so much, when my friends were talking to me, I was quietly counting the number of letters in their sentences.

After I moved to Canada, I thought it would be impossible for me to start counting the letters of English words; not only because I didn't know how to speak English to begin with, but obviously because the spelling added a new layer of difficulty. But I thought I got nothing to lose if I tried. As I was learning the language, I started counting letters again. Sooner than I thought possible, I was doing it in English.

Looking back at this I realized something tremendous: the reason I could calculate close to 40 letters in about 4 seconds was not because my brain had any extra qualities to it. It was because of *repetition*— nothing else. It took me months and months of overusing my fingers and toes before I established a formula in my head that allowed me to count the letters that fast. And that consistent repetition created a beautiful new network of neural pathways in my brain, which in turn generated the habit. With consistent practice, any skill can be developed and perfected. We can truly do anything we put our minds to, as long as we give the habit a chance, as long as we give it time.

But creating neural pathways, thus habits, doesn't stop at our own brains. It also extends to the brains of the people we regularly come in contact with, especially our children. The kind of experiences we create through the emotions we display— whether fearful, sad, anxious, peaceful, content, etc— help initiate and strengthen new neural pathways in their brains, particularly when they are at a very young age. What kind of habits do we want our children to acquire? If, for example, you repetitively yell at your daughter to clean up her room instead of saying it nicely, you are forcing negative neural pathways on her. As a result, she will start associating cleaning with a negative emotion, and she will most likely never do it just because she wants to. We heard many times that children whose parents force them to eat everything on their plate have a bigger likelihood of developing eating disorders later in life. Neural pathways develop in their little brains that associate eating with very negative emotions related to their parent's behavior, and they could end up having an eating disorder. We should always be conscious of what we repeatedly say, but most especially *how* we say it.

With time, patience and focused attention, our complex brain has the capability to not only create new habits, but also reverse habits. Once you come to terms that no amount of time is ever too much to devote when it comes to creating a better version of you, you are halfway there. After that, it becomes a bit easier to do the actual work: undo your unwanted habit by steadily taking your attention away from it, while putting your attention on a counteractive positive habit that will support the new choice. In a nutshell, it's as simple as that.

I'm aware that discreating a bad habit could be more challenging than creating a brand new positive one. Sometimes those neural pathways could be so strong they cause intense withdrawal effects, which keep pulling you back into the unhealthy behavior. It's very much possible to eliminate such habit, although more focused attention and will is required (and in some cases the help of a qualified practitioner). The great news is that unlike the rest of the creatures on this planet, we have the perfect tool to achieve that: we have a *prefrontal cortex*. The prefrontal cortex is the part of the brain that has the executive function; it is where much of our intelligence and problem-solving ability lies. As Dr. Perlmutter states, *"Unlike the amygdala, the prefrontal cortex allows for measured, careful responses to situations, giving consideration to various outcome possibilities and allowing for the evaluation of the implications of various choices."*

This is a valuable tool we possess and which separates us from the rest of the creatures on Earth. Once consciously employed— by THINKING before we act or say something we might regret— it can truly keep us out of trouble. Experts call this *mindfulness*. Being mindful is being focused on the present moment, acknowledging one's thoughts and feelings. By practicing this consistently you can build neural pathways between the amygdala and the pre-frontal cortex, so instead of overreacting when you're stressed, you can respond consciously.

Here is a diagram illustrating what happens when bypassing the pre-frontal cortex— in other words, when acting on impulse:

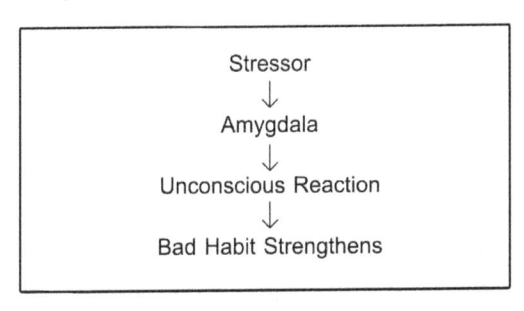

```
Stressor
  ↓
Amygdala
  ↓
Unconscious Reaction
  ↓
Bad Habit Strengthens
```

The following diagram illustrates what happens when we take control over the direction of our thoughts by employing mindfulness— in other words, when we *think* first:

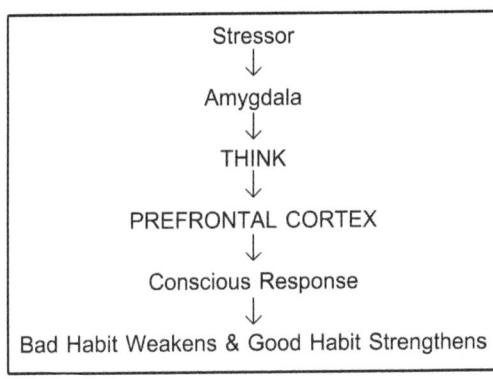

```
Stressor
  ↓
Amygdala
  ↓
THINK
  ↓
PREFRONTAL CORTEX
  ↓
Conscious Response
  ↓
Bad Habit Weakens & Good Habit Strengthens
```

You can see that by simply *thinking* before you act the whole process is deviated. Most— if not all— of this habit creating matter is based on the *think* (or being mindful) idea. It's where making life-promoting choices fits in. Once you ditch the bad habit in favor of a life-promoting choice, then sustain the new choice with focused attention and repetition, the old neural pathways weaken. This results in the bad habit gradually losing power over you. Focused attention is an important ingredient in this process, as it assists in the formation of the neural network in charge of the new healthy habit.

The brain is a very sophisticated organ, which makes it not so easy for highly trained scientists to completely figure out. However, our medical system makes incredible leaps almost by the day; ideas that only years ago were considered rather science fiction are palpable results today. Incredible discoveries have been achieved regarding how the brain works, with one top amazing realization being this: not only can we *deliberately* stop the brain's demise by repetitively engaging in certain routines, but the brain has the capacity of regenerating itself. Alex Schelgel, graduate of Dartmouth University notes in the *Journal of Cognitive Neuroscience*, *"Now that we actually do have tools to watch a brain change, we are discovering that in many cases the brain can be just as malleable as an adult as it is when you are a child or an adolescent."*

We are extremely lucky to be living in these times. The knowledge alone that is available to us makes the tremendous difference between stagnating and moving forward until the very end. THE BRAIN CAN REGENERATE ITSELF— do you realize what this means? It means that, regardless of age, it is wholly in your power to decide TODAY whether you start learning something entirely new; something maybe up until now you didn't believe it can be turned into reality. It means that no matter how old you are, you have the capacity of driving your inner most desires to the forefront of your thoughts and push them out into reality— by simply *making a choice and following through with it*. It means there is always hope.

And hope is a very good place to be in.

THE BELIEFS
— Habits of Thought —

When we think of habits, we mostly think of something we *do* such as smoking, drinking, or exercising. We often don't realize that what we *think of repeatedly* is also a habit. I would say this is the most deceitful of all habits because in some instances we're not even aware we're doing it. Habits of thought hide under various forms, one of them being what we call *beliefs*. Yes, beliefs are the result of habitual thinking and that makes them habits as well. They are the result of neural pathways formed over a period of time, and they can be either constructive or destructive. Further, these beliefs can also play a role in how easily one lets go of other unwanted habits and/or creates new ones.

The beliefs I'm mostly going to refer to here are not the ones hidden deep into our unconscious mind, the ones developed as a result of traumas and/or distressing events. What I'm referring to here are the beliefs people around us have been voicing repeatedly, and which we eventually took up as truths.

I'm referring to negative sayings, proverbs, mottos, concepts we consciously say, like *"Life's a bitch and then you marry one"*.

There are countless beliefs most of us grew up hearing and which we almost had no choice but to adopt. As children, we took over our parents', teachers', or friends' verbal legacies and robotically continue implementing these nonsense lies, passing them down to our own kids. I call them *default beliefs* because we accept them without questioning. We think they are harmless— that they are "just words"— when the truth is, the more we repeat them the more they put us on automatic pilot. As convenient as this might seem (giving up control and letting something else chauffeur us around) is not always in our best interest. Default beliefs will always take us in a default direction. That wouldn't be a problem if they were constructive beliefs, but that's rarely the case. Please answer this question quickly: can you state one positive saying you grew up hearing repeatedly?

Time's up.

Did you come up with one?

Aside from the ideas passed down from one generation to the next— such as the infamous *"You can't teach an old dog new tricks"*— there are also statements which, for one reason or another, we create ourselves and repeat over and over. A common one would be "I'm fat", when in actuality the person is not overweight. I happen to think that when a fairly fit person makes such a statement, it's offensive to the people who actually struggle with weight gain. Whatever their reason is for saying such a thing— whether it comes from the desire to be complimented, or they actually believe they are overweight and put themselves in a constant race to reach their own vision of perfection— repeating it like a mantra in time will have some sort of an effect. It doesn't matter if the statement is true or not true; repeating it over and over can actually turn around and create it in real life. *"Did you know that what you say about yourself has greater impact on you than anything anybody else says about you?"* explains Joel Osteen, Senior Pastor of Lakewood Church. *"Many people are overly critical of themselves, saying, 'I'm so clumsy. I can't do anything right'. 'I'm so overweight. I'll never get back into shape.' 'I never get any good breaks.' They may not realize it, but they are cursing their future. Those words sink into their minds. Before long, they develop a defeated mentality, low self-esteem and diminished confidence. Worse yet, those negative comments can interfere with God's plan for their lives."*

Beliefs act like filters that drive you and deeply influence your choices. Depending on how long you've been giving them your attention they can become so deeply ingrained, they successfully control you from within the back of the mind— big smirk on their face and everything.

You might have a strong drive and put in the time to work out regularly but if you have a belief that it's hard for you to lose weight because *"I only look at food and I gain weight"*, you will have a higher chance of giving up, or at the very least you will not fully get the results you want. The expression *"I only look at food and I gain weight"* is a belief I heard many women voice out during the time I worked in the fitness industry. Frankly, this is one of the most ridiculous beliefs I've ever heard, and I'll explain why. Unless a person has a medical issue (such as an underactive thyroid), nobody gains weight unless he/she eats processed foods on a regular basis and/or eats too much.

Let's take another example. A divorced, resentful mother, who always speaks spitefully about her ex-husband, concludes her little rampages with *"All men are the same"*. This might create a new belief in her young daughter that men are not to be trusted. As a result, the daughter might have a hard time allowing herself to be in a long-term relationship. On the other hand, she might choose a partner who will be the exact reflection of her own understanding of the acquired belief *"All men are the same"*.

If you believe you are an individual who lacks creativity or talents because you kept hearing as a child *"Nobody in our family is an artist, so go get a real job"* or *"You're too shy to be on stage"*, you might lock yourself in a job you despise and miss having an occupation you would actually enjoy waking up to.

And what's up with *"The joy of being a girl"?* I hear this over and over again from someone I personally know; she usually says it in front her daughter, when referring to her period. In a way, I can understand where her mother is coming from because her daughter has unusual painful cramps. However, the painful cramps really have nothing to do with the fact that she is a girl, but rather with the fact that she most likely needs a medical checkup. I can already see clearly the girl's attitude transforming, as she's slowly starting to act as if being a girl is some sort of a burden. Repetitively hearing *"The joy of being a girl"* in such a negative context might affect her future choices, actions, and ultimately experiences.

Sometimes when good comes our way, especially if it comes easily, what do we say? *"It's too good to be true"* or *"It's too easy, something must be wrong"*. We automatically disregard a possibly wonderful opportunity because we immediately put it through our personal filters and judge its validity. "*Life is a roller coaster*" is another variation of it. Just like a roller coaster, set in concrete and steel, life will unfold unexpected ups and downs. It's a deceiving habit we employ sometimes, when something good happens we almost immediately think that the opposite will follow. We put ourselves in a state of expectation, which is a powerful state— when we expect, we project that something will happen. Therefore, it's most likely that a "down" will follow and when that happens, we sigh with relief and nod our heads, *"I told you so. See, I was right!"* which only reinforces the belief that caused the very situation to occur.

It is truly a paradox how these persistent, inflexible ideas seem to latch onto our brains and have power over our minds, when in actuality they are complete lies. How can *"Once a crook always a crook"* even begin to be accurate? How can an idea implying that restoration is impossible, be true?!

It's odd how we complicate almost everything and at the same time we take important things lightly. Just because some guy woke up bored one morning and blurred out *"Anything that can go wrong, will go wrong"* or "*All good things must come to an end*", doesn't mean we have to be like sheep and keep "baa-ing" into it as if we're brain dead.

Here is another one: "*The mind wanders*". We think the mind wonders on its own, that we have no say in what it decides to think. When in reality, we do have a say— we actually have *all* the say because the mind is not something independent of us. The mind *is* us. Your mind is who you are, it is your true self. Therefore, it is *you* who decides. When you think your mind wonders, it only means you had temporarily disconnected from the present moment and let your ego step in. And the ego never comes alone;

it brings along its army of other negative beliefs, past negative experiences, worries, fear, bad habits...

Forget about *"It's too good to be true"*, forget about *"It never ends"*, or *"The rich get richer, the poor get poorer"*. Let's not feed these lies any longer. Let's be the generation that stops perpetuating negative sayings, ill beliefs, and rusty old proverbs that don't serve us. Instead, let's make a habit of voicing out— especially to our kids— confidence-building words. We do not have to stick with the old if the old doesn't have the capability to raise one's spirit to the slightest degree.

Old doesn't always imply wise.

Holding on to negative beliefs can be just as toxic to our brains as living in a polluted environment. Being aware of what's going on in our heads becomes one of the most important tasks we have as humans. Our every day choices, decisions, and reactions are based on what we habitually think. Aside from being the precursor of how we feel, our beliefs are also responsible for every action that we take as a result of how we feel. What we think and believe on a constant basis is what drives us to act a certain way, talk a certain way, react with people a certain way, even walk a certain way. In a nutshell, it creates our temporary character. Unless you take control and do a brush through of your recurring ideas, you might show the world a distorted version of you. Your character might have shades of frustration, apprehension, fear, jealousy, resentment, low self-esteem, even hate. You become more optimistic or pessimistic depending on the nature of beliefs you adopt. This, in turn, influence whether you will go for something you know in your heart you should do. You might have a burning desire to write a book but if you have a belief that it's close to impossible to break through in the book business, you might not even start writing.

So are negative beliefs hard to get rid of? Not when you understand this principle: just like you created a habit of smoking, or drinking a healthy green shake every morning, or exercising, you also started believing *"Shit happens"*. It's just a habitual thought. No matter how securely lodged in the mind, unsupportive beliefs can be eliminated once you are aware of them. But in order for a change in your belief system to take place, you must take some time to get to know your deeper self. Too often, our attention is hijacked by the every day distractions. We don't sit down and simply reflect on things anymore. Once you make the choice of bringing to your attention your recurrent ideas and beliefs, you're half-way on the journey of being free of them. It's like turning on the light on a thief that's been consistently robbing your house. Yes, that is exactly what negative beliefs do: rob you of creativity and willingness to move forward into achieving something extraordinary. Now that you know the severity of what's happening, will you just stand back and watch this thief revel in your possessions?

When it comes to nutrition and fitness— topics that claim a pretty large share of our attention— there are many detrimental ideas that people hold on to. All these ideas push people into creating certain habits, and in the end it's these habits that make a difference in whether one gets the results he or she seeks. Working in a fitness facility gave me a unique opportunity to learn what people take up as truths, particularly my fellow ladies. Aside from *"I only look at food and I gain weight"*, I've also heard things like *"Being chubby runs in my family"*, *"I have to train at high intensity in order to lose the weight other women lose without doing anything"*, *"Yeah, but she was always thin"*, *"I have to measure everything I eat"*, *"Lifting heavy weights turns a woman very muscular"*, *"You have to eat fat-free food to lose weight"*, *"Anything I eat turns to fat"*. Maybe some of these ideas you probably never heard before. Believe me, I was just as perplexed to hear that a pregnant woman took her baby out at 7½ months because she strongly believed *"Full term pregnancy will ruin your body forever"*.

While interacting with women verbalizing such ideas— despite some of them claiming that they were "just joking"— I realized those beliefs were, in fact, their truths; truths, which they were living by most likely without realizing. Looking back, I can easily see why some were struggling with losing weight even though they were dedicated to their routines, while others got the results they wanted easier.

So, before you go ahead and make changes in your eating or exercising habits, start by answering this question: what is your mind truly invested in? Think of the area you're looking to improve and find any unsupportive ideas that pop into your head recurrently. What negative concepts are you accepting that have been pressing on your brake pedal, making it harder for you to make a lasting positive change? What is it that you truly believe that makes you turn to your old ways soon after you implement a life-promoting change?

Next, answer this question: what is it exactly that you want to accomplish? Don't go for an "essay" type of answer, but clarify your goal in a few simple words. Once you have it, create statements that will support that particular goal. I'm not talking about creating affirmations that you stick to your bathroom mirror and read while brushing your teeth in the morning. What I'm talking about here are ideas that you consistently think about all day every day, until they become your beliefs. These statements should feel real to *you* but more than anything, they should be able to lift and empower you.

As you can see, these are 2 very simple questions, and it's exactly because of their simplicity that they can be easily disregarded. Very often I heard people say, "Of course I know what I want!!" But when asked "And what is that?" they couldn't clearly verbalize it. Personally, I spent years thinking that I knew what I wanted but the day I finally took a break and asked myself these simple questions, I had a hard time defining my goal. I realized my dream was blurred by junk negative beliefs taking up precious space in my brain.

Everything that you've been taking up as truth exists in your mind as a belief. Thinking that you must do at least 1 hour of high intensity cardio daily in order to keep the weight off regardless of how much you despise doing that, is a thought you kept thinking, which turned into a belief. What does that mean now? It means that if you don't stick with your routine, if you miss a workout or two, you believe you won't reach your fitness goal. Now you feel guilty, and feeling guilty means you are a slave to your own belief.

To various degrees, we're all guilty of maintaining negative habits of thought by feeding them back and forth to each other. Then again, regardless of how long you've been holding on to these lies, in the end they are still only habitual thoughts created based on the same formula as you created any other habits: by focusing your mind on them on a consistent basis.

Beliefs and personal truths are interchangeable: we believe certain things because we think they are truth. But what is truth, really? Truth is that which is true to *you*. And whatever is true to you, you believe in and live your life by. So ultimately, it doesn't matter what the truth really is; what matters is what you believe in. Why, then, not make sure your truth is one that serves you in a constructive way? Why not make sure that it serves you in being the best that you can be, that it supports you in fulfilling your destiny?

Why not make sure that what you believe in is something you would want your child to believe in?

Become consciously aware of what goes on in your head and you will eventually be in full control over the kind of habits you have. Before you know it, you will have developed a strong positive habit of thought and your brain— now on the kind of automatic pilot you want it to be— will start rewarding you with thoughts of the same kind. "*What goes around comes around*" doesn't only apply to things we do. It also applies to our thought system. Thinking positive thoughts brings about more thoughts that are positive.

Each moment comes accompanied by freedom of choice. This means that in every moment it's totally up to you to decide which path you choose. You and only you are responsible for the direction of your thoughts, and ultimately what you believe in. You cannot change how you started off in life. Sometimes even events that happen through life are very much outside our control. What you *can* do however, is choose the most direct path to your goal. Stop zigzagging with your destiny and avoid agonizing, unnecessary delays. Regardless of how the canvas of your life looks like in this moment, no matter where you were born, no matter where you are now, no matter what you're dealing with, although it may not seem like it you are and always will be in charge of your habits of thought. Because God gave you a mind and free will. Yes, sometimes the winds of life bring in unpredictable clouds. But are you going to mope around feeling unhopeful or purposeless? Are you going to allow those (passing) clouds hide your sun forever and settle, yet again, for "*When it rains it pours*"?

Or are you, instead, going to add a rainbow to your canvas, *"Grab the bull by its horns*" and boldly dare to *teach an old dog some new tricks*?

THE REWARD
— "What's In It For Me?!" —

Bad habits don't form out of nowhere. There is always an initial incentive, a reward that catches your attention. The established neural pathways in charge of your harmful habits always bring with them the promise of this reward— a temporary good feeling— which makes you want to walk that particular path over and over. In other words, it makes you want to revisit the habit again and again. Every time you picked up that cigarette, you did it for one reason alone: the reward. And the truth is the habit has never disappointed you— whether it was the comfort you were seeking or your piers' approval, your habit never failed in giving you the reward that you expected, every single time. This reward, although short lived, is what makes it hard to turn away from a destructive habit. You walk the path over and over to reach the reward once more, not realizing that the more often you do, the more defined the path (the bad habit) becomes. Whether you are aware of it or not, the reward is what ignites the desire to engage in a certain behavior.

When I was in university, I used to smoke. Even though I was taking Musical Theatre (which meant smoking was double as dumb because singing was my livelihood), I did it simply because it was the coolest thing kids were doing. But I clearly remember the first time I put a cigarette in my mouth; when I inhaled the cloudy smoke in my lungs, I felt so sick! In that moment I could've easily put the cigarette down and never think of smoking again. It would've been so easy to do! But the reward behind my action— to fit in— was much stronger. I wanted to feel accepted, I wanted to be "cool". So I kept trying, and soon enough I was hooked on smoking.

The same principle applies in reverse, when trying to get rid of a bad habit. In order to break an unwanted habit, you must find a real reason to stick to your decision; something important enough for which to give up the short-lived reward you've been used to getting. Knowing what it is you're going to gain, as the result of your efforts, is imperative to sticking to the process. Motivational speaker Ed Foreman says that when you offer something initially, people are more inclined to return the favor. This applies to our own person as well. You need to give yourself something for the efforts you're going to put in, otherwise you're more likely to give up.

When it comes to overcoming an existing negative habit, it's important to have a clear answer as to *why* it is you want to make the change. What are you going to gain at the end of this journey? You need a *counteractive reward* as an incentive to keep on the right track. As it is one of the most important components in the process of discreating bad habits, this counteractive reward has to be realistic and enticing enough for you to want to deviate from seeking the reward the negative habit was giving you— the more enticing the counteractive reward, the better the chance to succeed in overcoming your bad habit. A well-chosen reward is extremely powerful because it is what ultimately fuels your connection to will (power).

Something else I would like to underline here is that the reward your negative habit gives is usually short-lived, and it's almost always followed by shame and guilt. The positive reward, on the other hand, endures over time. It will keep its word in giving you exactly what you want, every single day.

An exceptional example I had the privilege of seeing in my late father-in-law, who was a heavy smoker for 57 years of his life. He was about 75 years old when a frightening pneumonia episode triggered his decision to stop smoking cold turkey. Nobody thought that such an ingrained addiction was going to be possible for him to give up, more so because other people were smoking around him. I have to shamelessly admit that I, too, expected that any day he would resume his lifelong habit. But weeks passed by, then months, then years, and he never, ever put another cigarette in his mouth. What impressed me most was that although he was heavily tested when second hand smoke was around him, he remained completely solid in his decision.

How did he do it? He didn't have the aid of those popular nicotine patches or electronic cigarettes; he didn't become part of a focus group or attended any seminars. He didn't even go to his doctor to let him know he gave up smoking! I'm sure his ego did not fail in shouting out to him that it's impossible to give up such a deeply ingrained habit. But he completely shut down his ego by being very clear and laser focused on his goal. His reward was to be around for his family as long as he possibly could. And because that reward was much more important than the reward the habit of smoking was giving him, it was powerful enough to support him in overcoming his addiction.

Your reward could be anything; a desired image of yourself, an idea, even a material item. There are no wrong rewards. You might even find that what truly motivates you seems juvenile, unimportant, ridiculous, maybe even vain. That doesn't matter whatsoever. It doesn't matter if you want to lose that weight because you want to feel better, you want to fit back into your high school jeans, or you want to make your ex's girlfriend jealous. If it's something that has the capacity to deviate you every time you're about to give into your old habit, it's gold for you. As long as it doesn't hurt anybody, the reason you lost all that weight, or gave up smoking, or stopped drinking soda is your business and your business alone. It doesn't matter why you did it. What matters is that you did it. What matters is that you succeeded in becoming a better version of yourself.

There could be many reasons you might want to get rid of your unwanted habits. Maybe you simply did the math and realized that you spent over $100,000 on cigarettes in the 20 years that you've been smoking— money that could've helped pay your mortgage or made you debt-free by now. Or maybe your doctor told you that your health is in shambles due to overeating, and that there is a possibility you will not be here to see your kids grow up, marry, have kids of their own. Think of who is most dear to you and put this on them. If your self-worth is not strong enough, if getting lung cancer and possibly dying is not dramatic enough for you to make a change for yourself alone, then— and I'm saying this as lovingly as I possibly can— use your dear ones as the reason to change. Do it so they don't have to experience unnecessary pain.

The following is my experience with my life-long habit of overeating, a habit I initially had many failed attempts in trying to overcome. Ultimately, I wasn't successful until I searched my mind for a reward important enough for me to stick to the process. I had to find something that could stand the test every time food was in front of me; a reward that, as I had to remember over and over again, would not fade in time and lose its appeal. Here is that story...

I always loved to eat. When I was growing up my parents never, ever had to say to me "Eat everything on your plate". I would eat anything I was presented with regardless of whether it was fish, meat, vegetables, fermented foods, and everything else in between. This, of course, almost always resulted in overeating. And when I say "overeating", I mean it in the "professional" way; not that I will ever do it, but I'm convinced I have what it takes to be a fierce contender in one of those eating competitions. (It probably has something to do with the fact that I was born under the sign of the Pig in the Chinese horoscope— ha, ha.)

The good thing for me though, is that I was always active— starting with ballet in my childhood and young adult years, then fitness and personal training after I moved to Canada. So aside from a few pounds here and there, my overeating tendency never really reflected on the scale. I never struggled with my weight, but I did struggle with the way overeating used to make me feel.

However, overeating and getting away with it was going to change in forties. Between moving with my family to a new place and taking on a tad too many projects at once, working out fell to the bottom of my to-do list. I was what I would call "normally" active for me (taking daily walks and stretching), but I slipped out of the habit of actually working out. The problem was that my eating habits remained the same. Although I eat healthy foods for the majority of the time (I got rid of my sweets addiction long before this happened), the bottom line is that no matter how healthy you eat, if you eat more than your body needs, caloric wise, you will gain weight.

Unfortunately, I didn't realize I was slowly slipping toward that side. Being at home engrossed in my work, I didn't notice the extra pounds sneakily adding up under the sweat pants and baggy t-shirts I was wearing most of the time. I was truly blind to what was happening to me. The idea that *I* could be one to worry about extra weight was so far from my mind, I was actually proud that I could eat more than my husband does and get away with it!

At a certain point though, I started to get glimpses of reality. One time I put on a dress I hadn't worn in a while and to my complete and honest surprise, I could not close the back zipper. I also noticed I had a little muffin top, as some of the shirts I loved and had been wearing for years looked as if their bottoms shrunk. Other unfamiliar sensations were creeping up, symptoms I used to hear from my clients when working as a personal trainer, like low back discomfort, strength gradually weakening, neck and shoulders tension, feeling sluggish... These were all issues I used to preach to others that they are easily avoidable, should one eat right and be physically active. Now here I was, not following my very own advice! My mirror was now showing me an image that was departing from the image I had been holding in my mind for years. And soon enough, I started carrying this nagging, persistent uneasiness about my body image, which became a bothersome backdrop to my every day life.

Sometimes though, we don't "wake up" and make a decision to change unless something pushes us over the edge, so to speak. What woke me up to my *growing* problem was when I had to literally force on my all-time favorite pair of jeans— jeans I've had for almost 20 years and which fit perfectly a little over a year before. After I eventually closed the zipper, my family and I drove to Toronto for a stroll on the Lake Shore. When we got out of the car, I noticed that suddenly the jeans didn't feel as tight as they felt at home. Thrilled, I tell Giuseppe "See, these jeans still fit me!" Then I made a joke, "You want to see a superstar's walk?" and proceed to walk wiggling my butt. And that was the moment my dear family let me know the reason my favorite jeans seemed to still fit: I guess the material gave up while sitting in the car, and now I had a large rip right in the middle of the butt region. My "superstar's walk" coming with a bonus of a pretty revealing behind must've been very entertaining for the strangers enjoying their walk on the Lake Shore. I was mortified at the thought of all those people having a really good story to tell at their Thanksgiving family dinner.

Only weeks later, a second pair of jeans had exactly the same fate. Now I find myself debating whether I should stop wearing thongs! I quickly realized my thongs were not at all part of the problem, but my overeating.

At first, I thought "How hard can it be to just eat less?!" Then I had my rude awakening: a birthday party would come (35 people on my husband's side of the family alone), then Christmases, Easters, Thanksgivings, first communions, confirmations, even the mundane dinners, and I realized I was a complete slave to my habit. Every single time food was in my face I would immediately and mindlessly proceed to stuff up my face. Then I would feel shame and painful disappointment for being so weak.

I realized that more than anything, this destructive habit was leaving an emotional mark on me. I finally accepted the idea that I might have a real problem on my hands, problem which was not going to go away unless I took it seriously. Even though I was only about 15 pounds past my ideal weight, I knew this was only the beginning. I knew that if I were to do something it would have to be *now*, before the issue got more out of hand. My overeating habit was not really threatening my health, at least not yet. But what I knew without a shadow of a doubt was that had I continued on that path, I was going to eventually feel the downside effects of this unhealthy habit. Even if I did get back to my normal workout routine, the reality is that overeating is hard on *any body* regardless of how in shape one might be. Based on numerous scientific researches conducted by doctors such as Dr. Sasha Stiles, a family physician specializing in obesity at Tufts Medical Center, overeating impairs bodily functions and causes biological changes that can lead to even more food cravings. Eating excessively not only makes one feel uncomfortable, but it puts constant strain on the entire digestive system, making all organs overwork. Excessive consumption of animal protein can lead to gallstones, weight gain, coronary heart disease, inflaming arteries, clot formation and heart attacks. It can cause congestion of the blood and lymph, suffocate cells and compromises their ability to manufacture proteins, which actually leads to lack of protein in the body. The excessive protein leads to a malfunctioning liver due to a high amount of toxins in the body from undigested foods. It can also cause kidney damage, pyorrhea, atherosclerosis, heart disease, intestinal deterioration, and cancer. Overeating reduces stomach acid levels, it can cause gastritis that could lead to internal bleeding and ulcers; it causes cells to divide faster, promoting cancerous growth because of the increased chances of DNA being damaged. Overeating sugary foods exhausts the pancreas, which leads to high levels of insulin causing blood glucose to plummet to hypoglycemic levels, damaging the metabolism and often leading to diabetes. Eating excessive amounts of food is considered biologically comparable to smoking cigarettes and air pollution, not to mention it accelerates aging.

Based on the intensity of my overeating habit, some of that would've eventually caught up with me.

Now, I understand that 15 extra pounds over the ideal weight seems like nothing. I probably could've tried to accept it as "normal" since I was in my forties; move on with life, think of more important things. But no matter how hard I tried to come to terms with that, I couldn't. And then it occurred to me to ask myself a simple question: "Why is it so important that I lose the extra weight?"

I was more than surprised to discover that my answer was a pretty simple one: because of the freedom that comes with it. I love feeling healthy; I love being able to jump and run when I play with my daughter, go up and down the stairs in my house as many times as I have to without feeling out of breath, being able to wear more than just the shoes I used to wear in my twenties. I love all those things! I just didn't know how important all that was to me until I brought it to my full attention. Finding my reward was my turning point.

You might wonder how something like stomach bleeding, accelerated aging, possibly even cancer did not convince me to make a change, and something so simple could. If you think about it, does it really matter? No, and I will explain why.

There could be many significant stresses inconveniencing us. We deal with them the best we can, and then they go, hopefully. Since their intensity is very high at times, we tend to put most of the importance on learning how to deal with these unanticipated stresses; which is a valid point— it is important to create a skill, a habit, of not letting unexpected high pressures get the best of us. But what about the "little" stresses? What about those small but constant, day in and day out worries? It seems their importance suddenly diminishes in front of the bigger pressures. These "little" issues we so easily disregard are usually deeply personal, some of them particularly intimate. They are the kind of long-term concerns that keep chronically playing in the background of our life day after day, 24 hours a day— like being persistently bothered by those 15 extra pounds that you gained in the past year, something you never had to worry about for over 40 years. Those seemingly insignificant 15 extra pounds, which are enough to make your entire wardrobe look like a bad idea. Those trivial, "it's normal when you reach your forties" 15 extra pounds, painfully reflected in that little muffin top you keep pulling your suddenly shrunk blouse over. We automatically consider these "insignificant" issues benign and tend to let them go, feeling secretly guilty that we had the nerve to even consider them. "There are more important things that need to be taken care of first", right?

Well, I arrived to the conclusion that there is no big or small stress but simply *stress*. In my book, ANY stress that stresses you out has to be taken seriously. It really doesn't matter how big or small the problem looks from a different point of view. It doesn't matter if it seems insignificant or spoiled or even vain to others. What ultimately matters is that it became a regular nuisance to you. Regardless of what it is, if it consistently disturbs you, it will affect your life negatively to a certain degree. Nobody can tell you that you shouldn't be concerned by it because nobody lived in your shoes, or in your head, to make that decision for you. When you think of it that way, don't those "insignificant" 15 extra pounds become an important issue? One worthy enough to make a priority and fix?

You might find it as a surprise to learn that throughout my whole life I never truly enjoyed working out. I always did it because I knew I had to; always dragged myself to the gym, dreading the thought that the next day I had to do it all over again. I actually hated the fact that my health and how I felt in general depended on something I almost despised doing. But something extremely interesting happened once I found my reward: I started to actually enjoy working out. I started appreciating that it invigorates me, that it makes me feel like I accomplished something good for myself. When my muscles are sore the next day, it's like a warm pat on the back acknowledging my hard work, determination, and consistent effort I put in creating such a constructive habit. In the end, feeling empowered because of the change in this one habit alone feeds my motivation to stay on the right track.

Don't get me wrong, I still love eating. But I realized my reward is much more important than eating excessively. When food is in my face now, I immediately think of which of the two matters most to me. As soon as I bring that to my attention— as soon as I *think*— overeating looks like a mindless, primitive action. So instead of inhaling my food, now I enjoy my food. Once I started eating the proper amount of (clean) foods and exercising regularly again, it didn't take very long before I lost those 15 pounds. (You can see before and after pictures at the back of the book.)

If your decision to eradicate a bad habit is fuelled by a solid reward, it makes all the difference in the world. Your health doesn't have to be at stake in order for you to want to make a change. Whatever your reason is, your reward is going to carry you through until your new positive habit turns automatic. It will be that anchor pulling you back when you're about to wander just a bit too much.

Ask yourself: what is the *real* reason behind your desire to lose weight? Did weight become an issue after you had your baby? Is it a health matter? Is it because you want to look better for your wedding? Do you want to fit into your old bathing suit? Do you simply want to feel better?

All the reasons above are equally as valid. At first, it probably sounds unkind to say that doing it to survive from an illness and doing it to fit into your skinny jeans are equally legitimate reasons. But as I explained earlier, any reason is important because *how you feel is important*. And the way you feel greatly influences life around you. Whether you want to lose weight because your doctor said your blood pressure reached life-threatening levels or because you want to fit into your old bathing suit, as long as it doesn't hurt anybody, is irrelevant. The bottom line is that the extra weight makes you feel bad. And when you feel bad— regardless of the reason— you're more or less constantly under pressure.

Think of a reward you would enjoy more than the short-lived reward the bad habit gives you. Once you decide what's truly important to you, once you solidify that future reward in your mind, make sure you find an effective way to remind yourself of it every time you feel the urge to give into the old pattern. If you decide that your reward is an improved body image because you simply want to look better on your next family vacation, you could place a picture of your past thinner self somewhere you can easily see it. Make it your cell phone wallpaper for example. It literally takes an instant to forget all about the new plan and give into the old habit of eating the wrong foods. But if the reward you're seeking is in your face all day every day, you're most likely to stay focused on your goal. *"Keep your eyes on the prize"* is truly the best way of putting it. You can do that by being more mindful, by employing the THINK part of the process. It is your prefrontal cortex at work, you most likely have it (ha ha), so make sure you put it to work. Dare yourself to use that bigger, human part of your brain, and prove to no other than yourself that you're more than just the host to a sometimes unreasonable, overreacting nugget: your amygdala.

No one can say for certain how long it will take you to discreate your unwanted habits and fully create better ones. But there is one thing you *can* be sure of: if you do not get swayed away by that unknown, you will succeed. Keep walking that imaginary path until you reach your accomplishment in real life. Do not stop until you look in the mirror and see the reward looking back at you.

Do not stop until you become your reward.

THE WILL
— Your Habit Predecessor —

It is not your will you must strengthen,
but your desire to discover its full potential in you.

Understanding that we have a will that can support us, especially through the tough times imposed by our detrimental habits, is imperative. A deep-seated harmful habit cannot be overcome without the assistance of will.

On the other hand, will cannot assist unless it is *allowed* to do so.

I used to believe that every person had their own will, which could be of various levels of strength. I used to believe strong willpower is absolutely necessary if you are to quit smoking, or overeating, or wanting to create a habit of getting up an hour early to go to the gym. I was always searching for new ways to strengthen my will and it seemed the more I was focused on it, the harder I was falling back into my bad habits.

Then one day I realized that all this nonsense couldn't be further from the truth. I realized the problem didn't lie in my "weak" will as I thought, but in the *obstacles I placed between myself and will*.

Will is synonymous with *strength*, *able*, *can*. It is the precursor of a positive action, the fuel behind life-promoting habits. We use it when we want to accomplish something constructive— I've never heard anyone say, "I'm going to strengthen my will to start smoking". Most importantly, there is no such thing as "my will", "your will", "his will" or "her will. Will is one, and it originates in God. Therefore, you can't think that your will is weak and not undermine Him.

Think of will as a boundless pool of strength that God extends equally to all of us. Although we all share it, it doesn't mean we each have a small part of it. (It would be like saying that if one million people pray to God, each person gets one millionth of His attention.) Its supply is unlimited and uninterrupted, therefore nothing we think or do can chip away at its ability to serve each and every single one of us fully and indiscriminately. Will is like a sacred, infinite reserve of supernatural power suspended in its own sacred dimension, humbly being there for one purpose: to serve us. Will— like God— is always there, predictably consistent. At any given time, every one of us can tap into it should we simply choose to.

However, even though we can never break our connection to it, will can temporarily fade in the background of our poor choices. This is what makes the unfortunate difference— the filters, the walls, the barriers that we place between us and will. These obstructions come in various forms, from negative habits and beliefs, to fears, to letting our irrational egos decide, to plain old laziness.

Why do I think it's so important, or worth the effort, to clear the path and let will assist us in overcoming negative habits? Why do I think it's so worth the effort to create a fulfilled, meaningful life? Because I did otherwise

79

and I know how it feels. I'm very familiar with being in the humbling place where I was counting the years I might still have to live. During the time I struggled with chronic habitual anxiety and panic attacks I used to think to myself, "I'll live another 50 years at the very most. Ok, it seems like a long time but once I'm done, I'm DONE. I'm gone, on the other side, where this kind of stuff doesn't matter." But it doesn't work that way. See, God gave you complimentary franchise in His will for a very good reason. He didn't give it to you to use it merely in this split-of-a-second life and be done with it. He gave it to you for much more than that. When you learn something and expand your mind, when you let will overpower your ego and your hindering habits, when you overcome pain by consistently getting up to better yourself, you do it for much more then to live a fulfilled life— you do it to advance your soul. You do it for eternity. Everything that your mind encompasses here in this life, you take with you. You won't take your house, your gold, or your money (the Egyptians tried and it didn't work, ha ha), but you *are* going to take the knowledge, the experiences, the learning, the wisdom. It all becomes part of the ultimate you, your soul.

It is not your will you must strengthen but your desire to discover its full potential in you. Once you know where your will comes from, it becomes the voice that overrules the chitter-chatter barking at the back of the mind— I call it "ego's noise". Ego's noise is nothing else but the result of a panicking amygdala and urges shot out by neural pathways conditioned to maintain a particular habit. The good news is that the more you strengthen the habit of remembering will, the easier it gets to silence the ego's noise.

When you don't deliberately clear your connection to will, destructive habits form by default. Conscious use of will, on the other hand, creates constructive habits. But you have to *know what you want*, understand *why* you want it, make a plan and follow it consistently, then the power of will is going to propel you forward. Despite of how deeply rooted your negative habits may be, once you focus on using will the right way, everything is going to become clear, and yes, even simple.

The following is a story about one of the most gratifying experiences I personally had with the power of will...

Since I was a child, I loved bedazzling my stage clothes and shoes. But at the time in Romania we didn't have fabrics already embellished or even the possibility of buying sequins by meter. In order to finish a bustier I was going to wear on stage, I had to ask my friends to collect the sequins off their mother's old dresses.

When I moved to Canada, I discovered the Swarovski crystal and I was completely taken away by the beauty of this element. I started crystallizing jeans, microphones, cake toppers, shoes, my daughter's water bottles... pretty much everything with a flat surface. I then became a Swarovski Branding partner, meaning I could use their official tag on my work. Once I reached this point, I thought it would be a good idea to take it to a different level and do something more out of the ordinary. After a few months of brain storming with Giuseppe, we came to the crazy conclusion that crystallizing an Indian motorcycle would be an interesting canvas to apply Swarovski crystals on. My thought was, "It will need what, 30,000, 40,000 crystals to completely cover it? No problem, I'm fast. I'll get it done in a few weeks!"

Of course, I had no idea whatsoever what I was getting myself into!

We leased the motorcycle and the day it arrived at our house, Giuseppe and I became speechless. We looked at this 9-feet long, 800-pound black beast and both realized this might be a far more out of the ordinary project then we initially thought.

After 2 weeks of working 8 to 10 hours a day, I had barely 500 crystals placed on it. By this time, I felt broken. The consistent crouching down to the floor to do the sanding, cleaning, gluing, then placing the crystals one by one, caused me terrible physical pain— I was having a hard time getting up off the floor to take a break. My hips were hurting, my low back was hurting, my eyes and mind were blurry from the glue, and I had a stubborn, extremely sharp pain in my upper mid-back which intensified at night, making it hard for me to get any rest.

With every crystal I was placing, I had more and more pain and resentment— just plain, negative emotions going through my mind and body. I COULD NOT BELIEVE what I had gotten myself into! What was I thinking taking on such a lengthy, exhausting project? When someone would ask me how the motorcycle was going, my answer was: "Did you ever hear of the Chinese water torture?" Then if they didn't know what it was, I would proceed to explain it to them in detail: "It's an ancient torturing technique where the victim is placed on a table face up, and there is a drop of water consistently dripping in the middle of their forehead. The forehead was found to be the most suitable point for this form of torture because of its sensitivity: prisoners could see each drop coming, and after long durations, as a perceived hollow would form in the center of the forehead, the victim was allegedly driven frantic. And that is EXACTLY how I'm feeling working on this motorcycle!" I would conclude. People would laugh when I said that and I would laugh along with them, trying to make it light for myself. What they didn't know is that I wasn't kidding. The next day, when I had to wake up at 5am yet again, with each little crystal I was placing it felt more and more like that little drop of water dripping away at my brain.

One particular morning I woke up early as usual. I sat down on the stairs in my garage and looked at this beautiful beast for about a half an hour, trying very hard to get my mind wrapped around how to complete it right, while keeping my sanity at the same time. "How am I going to do this? I can't stop now!" That was the moment I realized I literally put myself in a situation of no return. At this point, the motorcycle was entirely sanded down. I had only one choice: to go forward. I had to somehow find a way to make peace with what I was seeing ahead— and what I was seeing ahead was at least 9 months of work.

Believe it or not, I wasn't aggravated at the fact that it was going to take much longer to finish than I originally thought. It wasn't the fact that I basically destroyed a perfectly good paint job off a very expensive motorcycle. Or that I had to cover it in (only what I could guess at that point) tens of thousands of crystals, each placed individually by hand, in a puzzle design, using 6 different crystal sizes, with the smallest being the size of a pin head... This was something else entirely. It was a *mind game*. It became clear that in order to see this project through, what I needed more than anything was the right mind set.

But how do you get that?

Then I remembered something I heard a long time ago, a way of training the mind. In this exercise, the student is given a very old, dirty pot, which he's expected to clean perfectly regardless of how long it might take. The exercise is intended to create patience, and puts one in a meditative state.

I realized I had to stop thinking about my motorcycle as the "Chinese drop" and, somehow, change my perspective to "Cleaning the pot". I had to fully grasp a very simple, yet powerful concept: with every single little crystal I was placing, I was one small step AHEAD— not stagnating, not going backwards, but ahead. Instead of looking at how much I still had to do, look at how far I'd come since yesterday. I had to consider this experience as an exceptional opportunity to clarify my focus and strengthen my will (yes, at this point in time I still believed it was my will that needed help).

And I did. I gave myself no choice but to finish it and finish it right. I put my ego aside, let myself be broken down by the experience and be rebuilt back up. Then something absolutely amazing happened. As if I got a mental reset, my mind kind of shut off and opened up at the same time. I suddenly felt absurdly clear: I knew what outcome I wanted and simply went for it, without questioning the process. I felt transported to an ego-less state where there was no beating around the bush. A state in which there were no doubts, no detours, no delays, and no whining. A state where visions, very simply, GET DONE.

That was the moment I understood the true source of WILL. I understood and felt its connectivity to our Heavenly Father and the immense blessing it is to be able to possess such a remarkable, life-changing tool. Its presence was so undeniably straightforward and powerful, *it could not have come from me*. And it certainly needed no help!

From that point on this unique experience turned into something I now regard as one of the best experiences of my life. The whole process morphed from being a chore to being a remarkable opportunity of growth. I had no resistance whatsoever; I was calm, my mind was laser focused on the task. I actually felt wiser.

Interestingly, the pains in my body started to subside. I was sleeping much better and every morning when waking up at 5am instead of dreading, I had an amazing feeling of moving forward, of being in charge.

In the end, it didn't take 40,000 crystals to completely cover the motorcycle as I originally thought but 200,000. It didn't take up to 100 hours to finish it as I originally thought, but 1,500 hours. However, in my mind those numbers became exactly that: just numbers. They were there only to quantify my journey and make it so much more meaningful.

I like to refer to this experience as a privilege, an exceptional opportunity of growth— I had to quickly make a decision between remaining partially asleep or allow myself to be promoted to a new level of being. I had to either accept the experience and go upwards, or resent it and screw the whole thing up. In the end, my decision to simply move forward without complaining resulted in something extraordinary. The outcome was truly a one-of-a-kind.

Wonderful things can be achieved when we stop looking back, when we put our egos aside and disconnect ourselves from past failures, unsupportive ideas and beliefs. Wonderful things happen when we give ourselves no choice but to focus on progressing. When we make use of will in this way, we can achieve remarkable results. And the success could be exponential should we decide to focus on something we are really passionate about, possibly a dream we've been contemplating since we were kids.

There is so much in that experience that deepened my understanding about the mind, particularly about will. However, what becomes evident when I look back now is that, in reality, it wasn't as complicated as it seemed in the beginning. In actuality, it was all very, very simple. All I did was focus wholly on where I wanted to be, got up, and did it without complaints.

Do you think there is a difference between successful people and the not so successful ones? Do you think the very successful ones have some secret method or formula by which they govern their lives? Do you think that awarded bodybuilder isn't sometimes tired in the morning, doesn't feel like getting up to go to the gym for yet another dreadfully heavy workout? Do you think that straight A student doesn't feel like partying instead of burying himself in some library to study for hours? Do you think that 44-year old woman who decided to become a volunteer firefighter doesn't feel like sleeping in instead of waking up an hour before her family so she can do her demanding physical training? Do you think that millionaire who immigrated to North America with 10 dollars in his pocket didn't feel like eating out instead of always putting his money away so he can open that successful business one day?

Yes, they all feel like not doing the right thing sometimes. Some of them maybe even feel like not doing it most of the time. But they do it anyway. That is the difference. The winner does it anyway.

Will is the means by which everything was created up until this point, it is what continues to bring the technology and everything else even further— the WILL. This invisible force indiscriminately dwells in everyone. We are equally entrusted with this most valuable gift; it is part of the essence of who we are. Will is always present in our minds, put there for a reason. As it comes from one and the same place, my will and your will and everybody else's will is capable of creating equally wonderful things. The only thing that makes the difference is who chooses to tap into it and who doesn't. That is the only difference. It's not enough to have a goal, a plan, or the right skill in order to achieve something. It's not even enough to have all resources needed to accomplish that goal, like the right connections and more than enough money. What's most important is to "have the will", as we habitually say. Which, in my book, is having the awareness of where will truly comes from and clear its path of hindering habits.

Can you make a decision today— can you make a decision *now*— that from this point on you are going to use will consciously to any facet of your life?

As you probably noticed by now, I'm not a sugar-coater type of person. I absolutely despise beating around the bush. To me, that only means taking the longer way with a huge possibility of getting nowhere. So here it is: in the beginning, you may rebound to your old ways. It's imperative to remember that temporarily "failing" is very much part of the process. Don't expect to turn around and be a completely different person over night. Although I believe that is very much possible, most of us are not yet at the point where we can achieve that. So we have to rely on the step by step approach, which is great because it works.

When it comes to will, it's pretty simple. All you have to do is ask yourself this question: do you really want what you want, or not? If you do, then get up and do it. It's as simple as that. In spite of whatever it is you're feeling, get up and do it. That's the only way it will work. It's the only way anybody on the face of this earth achieved anything— by getting up and doing it. "But how long will I have to keep pushing myself to get up in spite of my not feeling like it?" you might ask. My answer is, "Until the new habit is formed". Again, nobody knows for sure how long it will take for your new positive habits to become automatic. But if you keep your mind focused on your desired achievement and not give up, you will succeed. You might feel as if your will is weak right now, but that's not the case. What is actually happening is that the path between you and will is not fully clear yet.

My will used to be so severely blocked by bad habits, it was borderline destructive. Starting from when I was a toddler up until my late 30s, I had an addiction to simple carbohydrates— sugary treats in particular. When I did get my hands on anything sweet, I wouldn't stop eating until I actually felt sick and sometimes threw up. Later on, after I moved to Canada, I would lie down on the couch in front of the TV and eat 8 or more butter tarts at once, no problem. Sometimes I would get a buttered white bagel from my local bakery, and by the time I was out of the drive-through that bagel would be already in my tummy. Then I would drive my car right back in the drive-through and get another one.

I did that 6 times in a row once...

Personally, falling into this downright addiction was not a way to soothe myself in times of distress— I wasn't craving simple carbohydrates when I was sad or bored. As a matter of fact, after my happy divorce at the age of 30, my addiction got even more out of control. I was binging on white breads and sweets all the time, regardless of how I was feeling.

Being so weak in front of unhealthy foods consequently made me think false things about myself. I started believing I was weak as a person, unworthy and unreliable. Even worse, I believed "I'm damaged goods", and that there was nothing I could do to change it. I truly felt a prisoner to my addiction and had tremendous guilt for being incapable of harnessing this invisible force residing inside my head, deciding what I should crave next and playing havoc with my health.

Over the years this issue grew considerably, until it became a permanent heaviness in my heart. It felt so massive and powerful, I remember distinctively feeling as if my spirit was somehow held back by it. I used to fantasize that if I ever broke this vicious circle, I could achieve anything in my life; that the sky would be the limit to what I could accomplish— if I could only beat my sugar addiction…

And I was right about that. Except when I did it, when I finally did break my life-long sugar addiction, an entire new chapter opened up before me. I suddenly realized I could do so much more than what I ever imagined. So much more!

You have no idea what you are capable of achieving, once you clear your connection to will. Every time you choose to simply get up and do it, you add yet another crack to the shell you've enclosed yourself in. The stronger you stand by your decision the clearer the path to will gets, and the more you come into our own. Then the easier it becomes to push away what hurts you and embrace healthy, enriching behaviors.

Once you decide to fully walk this path, don't forget that there is no such thing as "small accomplishments". Every single step forward— no matter how small— is a step that takes you closer to your destination. You are moving AHEAD. Don't let them pass by without your taking notice. The little accomplishments are the building blocks of a future solid habit that can hold the potential of turning your whole life around.

By sticking to your plan, the will *will* take you out of the proverbial darkness to places you've envisioned, and further. Breaking a sitting-on-the-couch-after-dinner habit is not only about the physical act of replacing it with a half an hour walk— it's much more than that. When you say *YES* to the walk, you say *NO* to the bull that's been suppressing you not only as a person, but as a spirit. You say *YES* to the infinite capabilities you were born with. You say *YES* to being who you really are.

Nothing can surpass will because it is your God-given tool to create wonderful things in your life. No bad habits, regardless of how deeply ingrained they may be, have enough power to stand in the way of your getting up and claiming a better life that is rightfully yours. Will brings the essence of who you truly are into the practicality of life. It facilitates your soul to come through and express itself— the clearer the path to will, the stronger your soul's presence.

THE KNOWING
— Know Who You Are and Where You Come From —

"God is inevitable, and you cannot avoid Him any more than He can avoid you."
— A Course in Miracles, Foundation for Inner Peace

Aside from understanding concepts such as the amygdala and neural pathways, the importance of will, beliefs and rewards that drive us, I would say the most important piece of information I personally had to learn before things started to change for me was learning who I truly am and where I come from. By that, I mean who I am at my core, before I came into the family that I was born in. Simply put, it is knowing we come from God. And because we come from God, there is a pool of infinite resources available to us at all times, should we choose to be fearless and tap into it. Knowing who we are and where we come from is, in my opinion, the ultimate piece of knowledge; it is what inspires us to easily make life-promoting choices. By understanding this single concept, one will get stronger in every way.

For a very brief moment early in my life, I had the immense privilege of fully understanding this concept and felt its remarkable outcome. Here is that story...

As I was growing up in Romania, there were many stray dogs on the streets, hanging in herds mostly around building apartments. These dogs would make people in the neighborhood feel very unsafe; not only did they disturb our sleep by fighting and barking in the middle of the night, but they also posed a real threat as they used to sometimes attack people coming home from work late at night.

I was about 11 years old when I decided to go to the movie theater to watch a popular Hindi movie (this was a movie I had been watching over and over, in an attempt to learn by heart the songs the actors were singing). As I was walking on the winding pathway in between two building apartments in my neighborhood, a large stray dog appeared on the corner barking at me so furiously, I could see his saliva pushed out forcefully through his big teeth. Being attacked by a stray dog was a fear we always had as kids, so without thinking twice I started running. That seemed to have angered the dog even more because he instantly launched at me running and barking, ready to tear me into pieces. Within seconds the dog was feet away from me, at which point it was crystal clear there was absolutely no way I could run fast enough to get away.

As I was running and crying in terror— realizing there was nobody around to help— suddenly the high panic in my brain turned into a powerful surge of energy electrifying my entire body. I instantly felt a kind of lucidity difficult to express in words— I stopped from running, turned toward the running dog, looked him straight in the eyes and let out a most powerful angry scream. While "attacking" the dog with what seemed to be an unworldly rage (wondering at the same time where that was coming from!), I quickly bent down to pick up a rock to throw at it.

But before I could even touch the rock, the dog stopped in its tracks, turned quickly, and RAN AWAY SQUEALING.

That memory is so vivid in my mind, clearer than any of my past memories. Looking back now, I realized that for that brief moment I knew exactly who I was and where I came from— which is not the daughter of two hard-working people from Galati, Romania, but the daughter of God in Heaven. That's the only possible explanation I could come up with, judging by the exceptional determination and confidence I felt in that moment. It's as if my entire being suddenly woke up (too bad I went back to sleep right after— ha, ha).

Who we are and where we come from is undeniably valid and beyond powerful. My question is, why is it that sometimes we have to be faced with a life and death scenario in order to tap into what we've been carrying with us from day one?

There are a few things that can block this innate awareness, one major reason being not knowing truly who one is. For some, their upbringing was conducive to knowing the reality of their origin, they were taught the truth right off the bat: that all of us, without exception, are God's children, filled with potential, strength, inspiration and most of all, ability to make life-promoting choices.

For others though (myself included), due to harmful beliefs we adopted at a very young age, knowing who we are could be a notion difficult to understand. I am somewhat of an extreme case when it comes to this subject. At a very young age I was faced with disturbing ideas, which instilled in me much fear and anxiety. These irrational beliefs were consequently the heavy foot stuck on my brake pedal and the reason behind my many challenges.

...Let's just say that the environment I grew up in was abundant in opportunities for spiritual growth.

As I mentioned before, my family is of the Orthodox religion. As much as our religion teaches about God, it also enforces that the devil is always going to be there, breathing right over your shoulder. *"The devil is always waiting at your doorstep— be vigilant of it"*, the priest in our church used to always say. *"He is so strong, with just the tip of his tail he can instantly turn this whole world upside down..."* What a notion to be learning from a person an entire community looks up to!

My parents were fairly religious people, especially my father. As he was also raised to believe that the devil is a step ahead of anybody, he was always on the lookout: took us to church regularly, taught us to pray before going to bed, and plastered our apartment with icons. There is no doubt in my mind that my father's intent was to be a good Christian. But his focus was entirely upside down. What he didn't realize was that by persistently wanting to protect his family from what he believed was lurking amongst us he was, in fact, giving more credit to the devil than to God. As a child I never understood, really, what the deal was with Heaven and hell. It seemed the grown-ups around me were looking up, praying to an unreachable God.

This constant display of fear made me grow up with a terrible contradiction: God is all, but the devil is closer. I was living with this unreasonable fear residing inside of me every single moment of my life— I was terrified of the dark and shadows, terrified of being anywhere alone even in the middle of the day, terrified of people screaming and other loud sounds, to name just a few.

I was— without doubt— the personification of the well-known expression *"Afraid of one's own shadow"*.

Fast forward... At 23 years old I entered into a 7-year relationship and marriage with a man who was dealing with his own bunch of internal/mental issues. Having to deal with his extreme, unpredictable behavior, as well as his constant soul-crushing insults, further intensified my fears and anxiety. That was also the time I moved to Canada and started a new life. In an attempt to *"best integrate yourself in this new system"*, as he liked to put it, he decided that I give up my music career entirely. He cut off my connections with everybody back home from family, friends, and music industry professionals. In an attempt to do just that— integrate into my new environment— I gave up on everything I was. For the following few years I worked in telemarketing and door-to-door sales. To top it all off, 2 years after I settled in Canada, back in Romania my 54-year old father passed suddenly.

Every unfortunate situation was taking my fears, anxiety, and negative beliefs to a yet more heightened level, making me feel constantly uprooted somehow. I felt like I was tightly surrounded by a mean cocoon blocking me from experiencing joy. I felt broken off from reality, as if living in a dream in which no matter how hard I tried to scream, no sound would come out. Even more saddening, I could recognize joy in others but was unable to grasp it.

In my tradition, divorce was almost completely out of the question. However, 7 years later it came to the point where having to constantly suppress who I really was began to have deep emotional and physical implications. Once again, I was faced with a tough reality, just like it happened when I was chased by that big, mean dog. I had to make a choice and very quickly: do I let myself be pushed over the edge and die?

Or do I fight back?

In the end, I chose to look him straight in the eyes and let the reality of who I was scream out. Once again, I woke up from an even deeper sleep and became in charge of my situation.

Through all my past adversities however, there were times in which all my negative beliefs and anxieties seemed to temporarily fade out. I consider myself truly blessed to have been given such a gift; a gift that pierced through my mind, revealing glimpses of a bright, uncomplicated and completely loving environment in which I could find relief. Those instances were mainly the times I was performing, and also messages I received through dreams and some other interesting experiences. It is those glimpses of truth that ultimately made me start questioning the validity of my fears and opened the door toward learning about the reality of who I really am and where I come from.

Performing (one of the 2 instances I mentioned above) has always been an opportunity of replenishment for me. Being on stage made me feel safe, it brought out the bravery in me. Up on stage I had a deep sense of belonging and was able to express myself as I wished. While growing up, I never really understood how the simple act of singing could do all that for me— I just knew I had to sing. It wasn't until much later that I realized something: that indescribable feeling of belonging came from bypassing all negative beliefs, fears, anxieties, and arriving in a zone where I was deeply connected to the reality of who I was. Something that meditation gives to so many.

My dreams and other interesting experiences on the other hand— truly a divine intervention— are the reason why I decided to approach the habit subject in this particular (spiritual) way. It is how I feel God would want me to approach it: if we are to successfully eliminate harmful habits that hold our God-given potential locked down, then it's imperative we understand who we are and where we come from.

Although the decision to share these particular details of my life didn't come easily, I quickly came to the conclusion that help came to me in this form so that I pay it forward. Once we learn something valuable, we must share with others. And in sharing, we also understand it better ourselves.

Fear is beneath you

What I'm going to start with here is an incredible experience I had years ago...

At this particular point in my life I'm experiencing the peak of my anxiety; I have panic attacks, which keep on going for days at a time. When that happens, I can't think clearly, I can't work, I can't eat, I can't socialize, I can't smile. My body feels strangely weak and heavy at the same time, and I have almost constant heart palpitations. And when I don't have a panic attack, I feel helpless and fearful at the thought that the next one is just around the corner. But nothing disturbs me more than the fact that I feel as if I had no access to my heart— the fear is so strong, I almost lost the feeling of love.

I get out of bed one morning and feel weaker than usual— I know I'm about to faint. Everything around me starts getting brighter and brighter until it completely loses its color. I feel I'm being pulled at an incredible speed through a narrow bright tunnel, leaving everything behind.

I'm not unconscious but very much aware of what is going on. I know I'm not in my room anymore but strangely, the newness of this place doesn't scare me.

A man appears and without saying a word he reaches for my hand, as if he wants to take me somewhere— it's Jesus. We arrive at a tip of a high mountain where He lets go of my hand and directs me to sit down. As soon as I sit down, my attention is swept away by the magnificent beauty unveiling all around me. This otherworldly place presented an elevated view of not only our entire planet, but the Universe itself seemed to be overseen by this peak we were on. I get an instant and profound understanding of the beauty and magnificence of life, which transports me in a complete state of awe.

As I turn my head to look at the steep valley opening down not too far from me, I notice something which telepathically gave me the awareness as to the reason I was there: I see FEAR in the form of a minuscule, insignificant, underdeveloped creature, crawling helplessly at the bottom of the valley— not in my heart, not in the pit of my stomach like I've been feeling since I was a small child, but AT THE BOTTOM OF THE DEEPEST AND DARKEST VALLEY THAT EXISTS IN THE ENTIRE UNIVERSE. And the only reason it's even there is because I decided to turn my head and look at it, because I decided to give it my attention. Otherwise, it would not exist at all.

This glorious feeling of lack of fear was rapidly expanding in my heart. I felt my being was naturally filled with immense love, knowingness, and graceful power. I felt the true permanency of life and the connection to one another— a state where fear is, simply, unacknowledged.

Next thing I know, I'm opening my eyes and see Giuseppe beside me gently slapping my face trying to wake me. He helps me get up thinking that I was weak but on the contrary, I felt inconceivably refreshed and at peace—as if my body got a reboot.

That was one of the most secure and unforgettable moments I've had in my life. The feeling of complete security that experience brought with it is impossible to do justice through words. It was, simply, magical.

However, even though I completely felt in my heart what God meant to convey through the gift He had just graciously given me, I didn't know how to mesh my new understanding with the practical side of life. At this point, I didn't realize that just like the habit of smoking or overeating, dwelling on fear (and having anxiety as a result) is also a habit we reinforce by our consistent attention to it. My amygdala, as well as the neural pathways conditioned to send me their anxious signals for so many years, were still in charge of how I was feeling.

As a result I felt strange, as if I was living as two different people: one serene and understanding, eternally connected to the highest power there can be, while the other half asleep, scrambling fearful in the dark.

On the other hand, this was the beginning of my understanding. For the first time in my life I could fully grasp the absurdity of being scared. I understood that my fears and anxiety were only volatile untruths spoken aloud by people who, themselves, were yet to awake from their own sleep. Once I was shown what fear really is— that it has no place in any of us— I knew that every one of us is watched over and loved with a passion that goes beyond our understanding. That the challenges we experience here are, to a high degree, our poor use of free will. And that can, sometimes, lead to horrifying habits.

The reason I brought up this point is to highlight how deeply beliefs can affect our lives. Regardless of how ridiculous, regardless of how childish they seem to be, they still have the power to hold one prisoner and turn to be the foundation of the choices one makes. As adults however, we're supposed to have a bit more wisdom and be more open to knowledge that can unveil the truth to us. This knowledge can come in a multitude of forms; from reading a book to listening to our mentors, or it can simply come in the form of dreams. But until we're ready to be flexible and accept change with all our hearts, whatever we were taught as children we regard as reality— no matter how far from God's truth that might be. I look back at that particular part of my life and I CANNOT BELIEVE how far behind that single lie was holding me!

You are love

A few years ago, I wrote a book of short stories called *Remember Who You Are*, which accompanied my original music album. In this book, I emphasize the importance of recognizing our origin and the myriad of capabilities we possess as a result. Just when I was about to send my finalized manuscript to be printed, I had an incredible dream— a straightforward explanation of the simplicity, yet profoundness of our being. This made me re-open my files and add this particular dream as a separate chapter. Its message is so clear and meaningful to say the least, that I thought it makes perfect sense to also add it in here...

A spirit in the form of a beautiful old man with white hair and beard cascading down his shoulders appears, and says he has something to tell me. The next moment, I find myself in the middle of a field. 'Look at this field" the old man says. I look around and I can see the golden beauty of a magnificent blanket of wheat, softly humming with each touch of the gentle wind as it allows the warmth of the sun to bathe its whole being. I have a strange feeling the old man can clearly feel my peace and tranquility.

A few seconds later he breaks the silence and asks, "What do you see now?" Then suddenly, a storm comes out of nowhere; dark clouds rush to cover the entire sky, and a torrential, raging rain starts coming down, ravaging everything in its way. Everything is happening in 3-D around me as if I'm watching a film on a circular screen. "What do you see now?" he asks again, with a peaceful expression on his face. I feel lost, almost in pain. I'm looking at this field, which one second was vibrating with life, and in the next second was lying lifeless in puddles of water on the ground. "I see . . . it's dead" it's all I can gasp through my frozen lips.

"Look again," the old man says gently. "In order to truly understand your meaning, you must bypass the physicality and see everything for what it truly is. You understand your physical world, as you barely need eyes for that. Now you are starting to understand your spirit by opening yourself up to it. But you will truly understand your life and its purpose when you let the physicality and the spirit come together as one.

I am here to tell you that you wrongfully stand between your physicality and your spirit; you have to come into the place where the fusing element— Love— is ready to do the work for you. Once you fully align with it, once you are ready to be vulnerable and trusting, to stand still with your arms wide open, your eyes knowingly facing it, welcoming the majestic light showering down on you; once you allow its vibration to melt the walls of sadness, grief, self-sabotage, drama, neediness, and guilt that you've built around you; once you let unconditional Love do its work through you, then you'll truly see and understand. You will see that this field is more alive than ever before. You will see its real beauty, which is incomparably brighter than the image your open eyes saw before the storm. You will understand that you and everything around you is eternal and can never die. You cannot keep yourself apart from that which you can never be apart from— you cannot keep yourself apart from Love."

A warm wave rushed and filled up my body from head to toe. I had no weight, no pain, no tensions— I was free. I knew in an instant this old man's very presence was the embodiment of pure Love.

You are a child of God and God is Love— *what do you think you are then*? Love is in everyone. Love is in you, in me, it is in your neighbor and also in the guy who gave you the finger on the road. It's just that many of us are not fully aware of it. We look around, rely on our eyesight only and quickly decide that what we see must be valid. But unless we make an effort to look at the world through Love's perspective, what we see with our physical eyes are simply judgments brought on by touchy egos.

The good news is that God never gives up in trying to get our attention. Whether through dreams, a song on the radio or just a random stranger on the street, He never ceases to try to catch our scattered attention. As He is not one to know failure— one by one we will inevitably come to recognize His truth. God crafted life in such a way that if we pay close attention, we can see the silvery trail of clues trying to catch our divided attention. Whether we like it or not, life pushes us to move forward, and sooner or later we hit our nose on the trail of clues and *get it*. Sooner or later we have no choice but to get it. It's the purpose of life to learn, to get wiser. In spite of our resistance, we always end up learning something.

You possess a powerful magic wand called *free will*, which is great. Sometimes though, due to lack of information, free will can be used wrongly; instead of listening to the voice of God, you can choose to listen to your ego. This usually results in detrimental choices and negative habits getting increasingly stronger because the ego is never reasonable. The ego will bring up all the negative emotions you have ever felt and chose to not let go of, and all the pain that comes with it. Now you value the ego, because the ego is telling you that your body is failing— see, you have pain now... And pain— in any form it might present itself— feeds your bad habits.

What sometimes makes the situation worse is that once you have struggle in your body, once you are a captive to any kind of negative habits, you may think your mind is broken. And what could be harder to fix than the mind?! You might think you're less, you're imperfect and always will be because, since you cannot overcome your negative behavior, your mind needs correction. But that couldn't be further from the truth. We tend to confuse mind with ego, thinking they are one and the same. But they're not. Mind is permanent and perfect because it is of God. The ego, on the other hand, is something we create when we let ourselves be overcome by stress, judgment, unforgiveness, hate... The ego and the mind are completely separate; thereby the ego can never touch the mind, although it can give the illusion that it does. Regardless of all that turmoil underneath, your mind is— and always be— as intact and as constant as it can be. Nothing can even begin to chip at its reality, simply because its reality is God. It is exactly because of this that you have the power to reverse any negative habits, despite how debilitating their effects may be. When you make the decision to be in charge and let go of your harmful habits— when you had enough of the bull— you are letting mind be in control. You are letting God be in control. And when you have finally got your *miracle*, when you have defeated your negative habit, you'll come into a strength you never thought you could ever have.

Arm yourself with the knowledge of who you are at your core, create the habit of thinking about it all day every day. Engage in activities that are conducive to reminding you of your true identity, anything that has the capacity to transport you to that point of understanding. Then hold on to it on a regular basis. Focus on who you are, focus on your inherent power— the one you undeniably have— and create neural pathways about that. This will weaken those neural pathways that have been lying to you for so long.

While you do this, your mind will slowly but surely come to light, while the ego and its pain will gradually fade away. The ego will come in, that's a sure thing. Possibly even harder than before at first. But you have to think of it as what it actually is: just a bunch of neural pathways that are simply doing their job. You want that! You want them to be strong, you want them to be insistent. Otherwise the new neural pathways, the ones in charge of your new habit, will not be strong either. You want them to be really strong. So when they resurface yet again— when you feel the old negative habit trying to take control— instead of letting yourself be crushed, get up and know that it's this very insistence that will eventually work in your favor. But you have to go through it, you have to— yes— accept it when it comes, you have to hold on to your knowledge. *Now you know what is happening and you are strong because of that.* You are where you are and that is the absolute only place from where you could go forward. Take a deep breath, lift your head high and, with a smile on your face and acceptance of what is in your heart, move forward in your own path.

I can't even begin to emphasize how important it is to know who we are and where we come from. If we had full trust in this single reality, there would be no need for any empowering seminars and countless books telling us what we should do— including this one. Once you trust and understand Who truly has your back, there will be no destructive habit that can't be overcome, let go of, forgiven and forgotten. You'll simply know that there is nowhere to fall. You'll know that there is no other choice but for you to come up as a winner in living life, simply because in doing so you magnify the expression of your true identity.

Maybe you are at a point in your life where you think that the *ideal* you is impossible to get to from where you are. What you should never forget is that although you might've not reached it just yet, what's important is that it exists in your mind's eye. What's important is that you can *see* it. And if you can see it, then you can focus on it consistently and achieve it exactly from where you are standing right now.

I believe at the end of the day everybody wants harmony and peace regardless of their actions, regardless if they admit it or not, regardless of whether they even know it or not. Whatever it is we do, deep within we do it because of a desire to get a glimpse of *that* feeling. But many times we go about it the wrong way, and that is when we hurt ourselves and/or others in the process. However, I reached a conclusion I can finally stay with because it is simple and the very thought of it gives me the kind of gratification nothing else could. *Knowing who you are and where you come from* is choosing to understand and accept the way God sees you: that you are truly a light in this world. It's choosing to be humble. Being genuinely humble is knowing that as a child of God, you are standing in the most powerful and favorable position yet have no need to show off. A position in which there is no need for drama and complications. You'll have no need to play games, wear masks, carry despise, or hate towards others or yourself. *Knowing who you are and where you come from* is living up to this inherent identity, which makes it easier to avoid harmful habitual behaviors.

So no more detouring, no more wondering, no more doubting, no more listening to the "peanut gallery", no more beating around the bush. What is it that you REALLY want? It might be to lose those extra 20 pounds, be free of that negative behavior or addiction. Whatever it is, know that the power is totally in your hands as to which path you take next. Are you going to look at yourself in the mirror and see the real you, a perfectly capable person who God loves above all else?

'Cause if you do, this whole creating/discreating habit business will be a walk in the park.

Chapter 2

YOU *CAN* TEACH AN OLD DOG NEW TRICKS

There are 2 distinctive points to creating and/or discreating a habit:
- The Moment of Decision
- The Being Steadfast Stage

The Moment of Decision is extremely short in its duration, in the sense that it could take a split second. Making the decision and genuinely meaning it creates a focused idea in your head as to what you want to accomplish. But you have to mean your decision with all your heart, truly be done with your old ways.

I mentioned earlier about my father in law giving up his 57-year long smoking habit cold turkey. He was a pretty quiet man who didn't voice his inner battles, so nobody in our family really knows how long it took him to beat his habit— nobody knows when he actually stopped having the urge to smoke. But I believe his moment of decision, fueled by his desire to be around for his family, was extremely powerful.

Once you honestly want to make a change, there is one thing you have to keep in mind: now that the decision is made, you took a huge step forward. Now that you've made the decision, you've taken control and confronted the negative in your life— you've declared your independence. This moment of decision is so powerful, it will illuminate the direction to your goal; a path on which you should start immediately and without hesitation.

The Being Steadfast Stage is the actual duration it takes to eliminate the unwanted habit (or create a new positive one). That initial glorious moment of decision has no resolution unless you keep steadfast in your choice.

Due to its personal aspect, the length of the being steadfast stage cannot be predetermined. However, if you simply trust the process despite not knowing how long it will take to see results, in due course you will reach the point where the negative habit will have no authority over you anymore. This stage is the period of time in which your amygdala, as well as the neural pathways in charge of the negative habit, will try full force to pull you back into your old ways and take control of your direction yet again. But relapsing along this way— although better to be avoided— will not compromise getting to where you want. As long as you keep focused on your reward and persistently get back on track, the unwanted habit will gradually weaken.

The following are 5 steps you can use as a guide when working on your habits; turning these steps into a routine will solidify the process in your mind. The first 3 steps help clarify what habits you want to rid yourself from and define your goal. The last 2 steps help speed up the process. These steps are:

1. Identify the Negative Habit
2. Eliminate The Triggers
3. Create a Positive Counteractive Habit
4. The *Put In A Dent* Technique
5. Develop the Master Habit— GET UP

1. Identify the negative habit

When it comes to nutrition and fitness in particular, it's not that hard to pinpoint your hindering habits— you know if you have a habit of exercising regularly or not, you know whether you overeat. Sometimes though, because habits happen gradually, it can be difficult to realize what's really happening until it becomes evident in some way. This happened to me not too long ago, when I gained those extra 15 pounds. It might sound pathetic but I honestly didn't realize I was gaining weight until my pants actually ripped open. I look back at pictures from that time and I'm staggered to see how obvious it was that I was gaining weight; meanwhile I didn't think I was.

Even if you think you know yourself, it's always a good idea to take some time to dissect each aspect of your life: your diet (meaning what you eat, not an actual diet), your level of fitness, your recurring thoughts, what you normally say, etc. Having a closer look at your emotions could also give you clues as to what's hiding from your awareness. If you find you're not at peace, if you have unexplainable anger, irritation or even just a slight uneasiness, ask yourself why. Emotions like this don't just show up out of the blue. Once you know what's bothering you, try to find what excuses you're making to not take control of this situation. Be honest with yourself, and most importantly accept the reality that you might be in error about it. In accepting it, you own it— now it's yours to do what you wish with it: keep it, or get rid of it.

So what's the first bad habit you're going to tackle now? Write it down, and make this its death sentence.

2. Eliminate the triggers

Think about what triggers perpetuate your bad habit and eliminate them at once. Are there unsupportive items in your house, your purse or in the drawers at work, that tease and trigger your urges? Collect them and put them in the garbage. Do you normally pass by a fast food drive thru on your way home from work, when you're hungry? Maybe starting tomorrow have a healthy snack handy, and change your route for a while.

Eliminating your triggers works really well, especially when you're looking to improve your eating habits. Although it's an action taken at a superficial level, something as simple as removing all processed foods from your kitchen or changing your route from passing by your favorite bakery, can help with keeping yourself on the right track.

3. Create a positive counteractive habit

One of the best ways to counteract those little neural pathways in charge of your bad habits is to create new ones in charge of a positive behavior. For every bad habit you want to get rid of, think of a counteractive positive habit that you can fall back on when you feel pulled toward your old ways. By switching your focus on a positive behavior, you will not only weaken a bothersome habit but will end up with a constructive, life-promoting habit in the process. Consistently focusing on a counteractive habit will act as a distraction from the old habit— and distraction is a *powerful* thing. Distraction is paramount in being successful at overcoming bad habits.

I understand fully how it feels to be like a programmed robot. I know exactly how it feels to be torn apart between knowing exactly what I should do yet not be able to find the strength to actually do it. What I noticed though, is that the more I was focused on my negative behavior and how to overcome it, the harder it was to actually do it. I could not get any relief whatsoever; on the contrary, it felt like the issue was becoming worse.

Things will most likely not improve if you focus on the problem. It's important to know what it is that's hindering you but once you're clear as to what you'd like to change, take your attention away from it. You want to weaken those old neural pathways in charge of your harmful habit, and the way to do that is by consistently distracting yourself with a new positive behavior and the reward is going to bring you. You want to create new neural pathways in charge of the new behavior, and you want to nourish those initially fragile threads of hope as much as you possibly can by giving them your undivided attention.

As soon as the bad habit starts creeping up distract yourself. Shift your focus. The old neural pathways that usually turn you into a wind-up toy and make you reach for comfort food will do their job perfectly and try to pull you back into your old ways. But here is where you have an opportunity to employ the human side of your brain, your pre-frontal cortex. If, let's say, your tendency is to eat when you're stressed or anxious even though you're not hungry, before you reach for the food stop and immediately switch your focus on your counteractive positive habit. If you are hungry on the other hand, make a conscious decision to reach for a healthier choice. Always make sure you have a snack/meal containing protein, carbs and good fats, and you'll notice that your desire to have junk diminishes substantially, even goes away all together.

Here is another example. Let's assume you suffer from insomnia induced by negative internalizing before going to bed. Your strong neural pathways are doing their job brilliantly, persistently reminding you of your problems. Let's also assume you have been thinking of meditating lately because you know it helps rest the mind, but you just haven't found the time to start it yet. Well, here is your chance. What you need to do is create a new behavior in your brain: every time you get worrisome thoughts think *meditation,* and make a consistent effort to clear your mind. Make meditation the distraction from your negative internalizing. Meditation teachers suggest not lying down when mediating, as you will most likely fall asleep. However, in this particular case you don't have to worry about that— you *want* to fall asleep. In time, you will create a new habit of clearing your mind, which will help you rest better and also introduce you to meditation on a gradual basis. Once you start seeing positive results take place, you might even decide to make meditation part of your daily routine outside of the times you go to sleep at night.

There are many good subjects from which you can choose to distract yourself and create your counteractive positive habits. You could take singing lessons, read, play music, go for walks or jogs, dance, clean your house, call a friend instead of texting (not to complain though), watch inspiring movies, learn how to sew, take an interior design course, learn how to paint, take a film scoring course, take pictures, become an aerobics instructor, learn how to knit, read your Bible, volunteer... There are so many creative activities to choose from and express yourself. Ideally, this distraction/new habit should put you in a peaceful and creative state. You just have to find what you are genuinely interested in and start doing it, even if it's minimal in the beginning.

Now you have a plan. The following steps will help you accelerate the process of eliminating your unwanted habits. As you move forward in this process, you will start seeing glimpses of your desired result come to reality. It's these small but crucially important victories that are going to motivate and support you even further.

4. The *Put in a Dent* technique

Intention is very powerful. To be able to create an addictive behavior just by simply putting our attention on it, we must be pretty able indeed.

When you combine intention with visualization though, you take this process to a whole different level. Visualizing long enough creates emotions; try to visualize you're about to get fired, and you'll feel worried and insecure. Now visualize going back into your childhood memories to the time when you opened up that Christmas gift you always wanted, and you will feel a familiar warmth in your belly.

Same applies to habits. We know that once a habit is automatic, something very tangible is already formed inside the brain: a cluster of neural pathways. This network became part of your body almost as much as your right arm is part of your body: it is there, it exists, it's physical. But even thought that can make one feel like the negative habit is in control of the gas pedal, it is only because of a temporary exchange of command— you gave the control to the wrong habit. Despite that, you are still in the driver's seat and in charge of the brake pedal; one effective way of using it by visualizing that you're putting a dent into the neural pathways in charge of your unwanted habit.

For example, let's say every day after having lunch you have a craving for something sweet. First, remember that it's those little neural pathways in the brain that are sending you the craving signals. Next, visualize putting an actual dent into them, and immediately shift your attention on having a healthier sweet (such as a piece of fruit or a small piece of dark chocolate). The beauty is— and I'm repeating myself here to reinforce this very important idea— as soon as you have the healthier snack, your craving for simple carbohydrates will most likely vanish. If in the crucial moment in which the amygdala and neural pathways start freaking out you stop for a second instead of giving into your bad habit, you give yourself time to switch the direction of focus. Remember the *think* part of the equation, or mindfulness, I mentioned earlier. Visualize that every time you reject to be a slave to your negative habit and choose to make a life-promoting choice instead— every time you choose to *think* before you act— you're putting a dent into the old neural pathways. This is making perfect use of the prefrontal cortex; by giving it time to take over the information and process it, you start breaking the cycle of something else being in charge of your actions.

As you work towards your desired goal, this dent will get increasingly larger, until the old neural pathways are severed in real life. Experts say that they will never completely go away; however, they will eventually weaken enough to come off the autopilot seat. Just make sure that at the same time you have your counteractive positive habit ready to take its place.

You feel like grabbing the nutrient empty desert? Think instead— do you really want that? Once you bring to your conscious attention the real harm that "treat" may cause, you will find it easier to make the right choice and pick a fruit instead. Every time you feel the old habit is about to take over imagine putting a dent into those neural pathways. Then distract yourself by shifting your attention on the new positive counteractive habit and its reward.

5. Develop the Master Habit— GET UP

Let me explain by saying this first: you do not need extra brain cells to succeed— you just need to GET UP. If you expected a more elaborate answer or some secret formula, I'm sorry to disappoint but I really don't think one exists. Of course, by getting up I don't mean it only in the literal way— I mean to rise up in front of whatever or whoever it is that restrains you. Whether you want to start exercising 15 minutes a day, stretch before going to bed at night, be more compassionate, drink enough water, move more, connect with your friends more often, have quality time with your child, drink a healthy shake regularly, get up 30 minutes earlier each morning so you can fit in your daily jog, write your new book or learn a new skill— whatever it is you want to achieve, you have to make that initial step to *get yourself up*. Get up every time your bad habit proceeds to wedge you down yet again. Get up every time *you know* your bad habit is keeping you from reaching your potential.

Rising up in spite of anything that's going on outside or inside of you requires self-discipline, a key ingredient when it comes to succeeding in any endeavors. It truly is very simple. Coming from someone who had a wagon of bad habits and broke loose of them (at least the most damaging ones), I can tell you that all I did was GET UP CONSISTENTLY.

I got to this simple answer after a while of dragging myself from the couch to the floor to do my stretches before going to bed at night. The hardest part was not the actual stretching, but to get my butt off the couch. That was the most difficult thing to do. Once I was on the floor stretching and my body started feeling better, I found no reason to stop doing it. But first, I had to get over the initial hurdle of getting up in spite of not feeling like it.

Every time you get up and choose to make a life-promoting choice— in spite of your not feeling like it— you force your way through the heavy layers of clouds that have been holding you back and tap into the magical power of will. The more you rise up to attend to your own personal needs despite anything that tries to hold you down, the clearer your connection to will; then the closer you get to the reality of who you are.

Absolutely any habit you want to create or discreate starts with getting up, both literally and figuratively. *Get up in spite of anything*. Now, that's the habit you want to create! Once you're up, you're up— you took the most important step. Now you're ahead of the game.

This is the remarkable outcome brought on by the habit of getting up, and that is why I decided to crown it as the Master Habit. Once this habit becomes automatic, you'll find that any habits you choose to adopt from this point on are easier to create.

We were given the remarkable ability to create neural pathways, thereby create any habitual behavior we wish. Imagine these neural pathways as little robots ready to take your orders; they can't decipher whether those orders are supported by your conscious willing or if they were created by default. They can't tell whether those orders are going to be life-promoting or not. All they know is how to wonderfully execute them to the tee. So take advantage of that. Take one little nasty habit at a time and smash it on the floor by creating a new positive one. Start on ONE habit today— a small one. Think of the smallest ambition you have and bring it to life.

Perhaps you want to brush your hair before going to bed— you know, brushing your hair massages the scalp and improves circulation. Not only will you end up with better looking hair, but you will feel better as well.

Stretch your hip flexors for 1 minute before going to bed— tight hip flexors, which occurs due to prolong sitting, is one of the major causes of low back pain; in many cases stretching can alleviate that discomfort.

Before going to bed at night, read the spiritual material of your choice and fall asleep with peaceful thoughts— scientific studies show that what we think before falling asleep gets picked up by the subconscious. The time just before falling asleep is the perfect occasion to purposely send the subconscious positive ideas. Then, depending on your consistency of practice, the subconscious does its magic and brings it to reality.

Drink a small glass of water with lemon upon waking up— it hydrates your system and gently detoxifies your liver.

Next time you're at work and need to go to the toilet, stay there an extra minute to clear your mind and release some of the accumulated stress, or stretch your hip flexors if you've been sitting a lot.

Turn off your mobile phone at 8pm to reduce some of that EMF pollution gallivanting through your body, playing havoc with your brain and energy levels.

After you brush your teeth at night, take 10 seconds to look in the mirror and say something positive to yourself— to build up self-worth and confidence.

Anything, anything at all that's positive, no matter how small and insignificant you might think it is, WILL have a constructive impact on your life in the long run.

EVERYTHING ADDS UP.

Take the time to get to know yourself, pay close attention to you as a habit machine. One of my favorite things is trick myself into doing something I would not normally do. For example, when I sit down to write on my laptop, I never sit close to my phone (yes, I still have one of those old landline home phones). I know myself too well; I know that if I make myself too comfortable in front of my computer, not even the sharp, nagging pain in the middle of my back would force me to get up because I'm a confirmed workaholic. So I work as far away from my phone as possible, this way when it rings I'm forced to get up and run.

Now here is an opposite scenario: I want to create a habit of drinking more water, but I know for a fact that once I start working I will not get up to drink. In this case, before I get to work, I put a big glass of water beside me.

The times when your mind has a chance to wander— such as when you're driving— is a great opportunity to distract yourself from falling into your old automatic pilot. Let yourself drift into your favorite music, listen to your favorite speaker, listen to empowering CDs, or even your favorite radio station. Use the time that you're driving to soothe yourself emotionally. If someone cuts you off, be mindful and don't jump to conclusions, start swearing and put yourself in a negative emotional state. Consciously try to create a habit of thinking differently. Maybe say to yourself *"... all this is, is a bunch of little neural pathways that I've been strengthening myself. I alone am the one who can put a dent into them and eliminate the habit. That person is someone just like me— maybe they are overworked, tired, in a hurry to get to their families; maybe they are hungry or have a hard time paying their bills. Maybe they have a loved one in the hospital or lost a friend to a devastating disease. Maybe they suffer from insomnia, or obesity, or diabetes, or migraines, or allergies. Or maybe they just have to pee really bad..."* Yes, there is always a possibility that that person did cut you off just to spite you because you were, maybe, driving the speed limit. But is verbalizing it worth bringing out the worst in you? Forgiveness is one of the most powerful tools God gave us— develop a habit of forgiving, and you'll be more at peace in general.

Switching your focus repetitively strengthens the habit of getting up, your Master Habit. In time you will create new empowering habits. Again, nobody can vouch as to how long it will take to reach that point. That is why it's imperative to remember something I purposely mention frequently throughout the book: keep practicing and don't expect a change overnight. As a matter of fact, things could get slightly worse in the beginning, which is unfortunately where many get stuck. But just because you don't yet see results doesn't mean the change is not set in motion and happening already. The only thing required of you in order to succeed is to keep getting up. Know that even though you might not see a difference yet, with every single time you consciously switch your focus, you are a little bit ahead from where you were a moment before. Reason being, the instant you initiated your good habit pattern, you started the birth of brand-new neural pathways. These new neural pathways are weak in the beginning. They can't act on your behalf just yet and so they desperately need your help. Your job is to repetitively switch your focus from the negative habit to the new positive one. The more consistently you support the new neural pathways, the less in control the old ones will be.

Chapter 3

THE POWER OF LITTLE STEPS

The little steps are vitally important when it comes to the process of creating or discreating habits. They are the foundation of the *being steadfast* stage I talked about in the previous chapter, and they represent the journey to your goal. I can almost hear you yell, *"Screw the journey, GIVE ME THE DESTINATION!"* Don't worry, I'm not going to preach, *"It's about the journey, not the destination"* because I personally don't buy that. I wonder if the person who came up with that idea experienced years of anxiety, extreme financial lows, or went through a crippling addiction. We like saying things like that sometimes, to sound wise. When, in reality, I think many of us wished this theory were false. Yes, I want to reach my destination and enjoy the results of my efforts NOW. I don't want to be stuck for days, weeks, or 20 years traveling toward something! I want to GET there. I want to BE there. And what's wrong with that? I say absolutely nothing. I say *"It's about the journey not the destination"* is just another one of those traps we keep getting our toes caught up in, to justify failure. In fact, it's brilliant because we easily accept it and makes none of us wonder of its validity.

It's about the journey not the destination" makes it OK to be stuck on a slow commute to one's destiny.

It's all right to want things now, no reason to feel guilty about it. It's human nature! It's our inner fire driving us forward. Wanting something now is not the culprit here— it's *how* you go about trying to get things done that makes the whole difference. It's about the approach you take to make that dream a reality that makes the difference between reaching your goal or being stuck getting to it. Are you going to choose a bumpy, cheap ride, by maybe doing the same thing over and over again and expecting different results? (which is Einstein's definition of insanity!) Or, are you going to embark on a smooth jet by clarifying your goal and create some good habitual behaviors to support it? Want it now— nothing wrong with that. The truth is that it *can* happen now, but you have to be patient and trust. This might sound contradictory, but I say it's not. As long as you have a clear image of both your existing unsupportive habits and the new constructive ones you wish to adopt, then follow the steps with patience, things are going to change. And yes, it can happen as fast as in the next moment of now.

It's very much possible to get off that detouring road but you have to be honest with yourself, you have to be willing to self-assess objectively. When you look at the bad habits that keep you from being your best, don't feel sorry for yourself— that makes you weak and keeps you from moving forward. I remember that feeling victimized was one major emotion I used to have when I was going through my sugar addiction. As I was reaching deeper and deeper into the wholesale box of cookies (at the same time knowing very well that that very action was going to hurt me), I felt more and more a puppet to my habit. I felt powerless, a victim in the most accurate sense. What I didn't know at the time was that just as I willingly put myself in that very predicament it is also in my power to get myself out of it.

Get yourself to the point where you had enough of everything that turns you into a victim. Thinking that way shoots you straight out of the powerless zone, and then you can begin to move forward. Create a habit of listening to the right voice in your head— the one that's annoyingly right (I'm sure you know what I'm talking about). Claim your power back by taking full responsibility. You can't be crying that someone or something else caused it all for you and expect to be in charge at the same time. You have to take responsibility. So your husband keeps buying potato chips. That doesn't make it *his* fault that you ate a whole bag before going to bed, right?

Want it now, nothing wrong with that. The desire to succeed in living life to the fullness of your potential should always be underlined with a sense of urgency. Not only because it will make you feel great, but because it will inspire others in the process as well— starting with the most important ones in your life, your kids. The world would be a much better place, for real, if more of us followed our dreams. But I don't believe we get there by forcing ourselves to "enjoy the journey". I believe we get there by making a conscious effort to be patient and repetitively taking the necessary steps. The sense of urgency to achieve any goal should not hinder the patience we need in order to get there. The sense of urgency is there to keep us awake and focused while going forward.

I'm not going to preach to you to enjoy the journey, but I am going to ask you to have patience. This is where your little steps come into play. In order to successfully eliminate a harmful habit, change your eating habits or follow a regular fitness routine, you need to take the necessary steps and have patience in doing so. Unfortunately, this is where many of us get tangled: we get discouraged in front of the unknown distance presenting itself ahead of us. Then if we do make the choice and initiate the change, somewhere along the way we lose faith in the littleness of our steps and lose the patience to continue. Do not be fooled by the word "little" though. Your steps might seem puny, but the reality is that they have tremendous power. Would you like to know why? Firstly, because no matter how small they may be, they take you *forward*, towards your goal. It's simple math: regardless of the distance between the starting point and the finish line, once you depart and keep going, you are instantly closer to completing the race.

Secondly, because *you are not going to give up*. There is nothing that can stop you, there is nothing that can make you go back, because now you understand that regardless of how slow you may be moving forward, you are on your way there. It's as simple as that. All that is required of you in order to reach the finish line is to keep going. You might feel weak at times, you might get angry for having put yourself through such dreadful process, you might even fall occasionally. But all that doesn't matter because you will— simply— keep getting up.

Meaningful acts get accomplished when you get up and do something about it. You can't expect to lose those unwanted pounds if you don't take the time to create a habit of eating healthy and being more physically active. By creating new positive habits that are supportive of your dream, you turn it into a realistic possibility.

No matter how big or small your unwanted habits are, you created them based on this simple formula: little by little. And this is exactly how you can also successfully discreate them: little by little. The same formula applies when you want to create positive habits as well. The only difference between habits, whether it's being a couch potato or doing Tai Chi, is the length of time it takes to undo or create them. This length of time cannot be foreseen, as it's personal: one person might take 3 days to completely overcome a bad habit, while someone else might take 21, 60, or even 120 days to reach the same result. That's why having patience is crucial. You might not know exactly how long it will take to get rid of your habit, but what you do know is that each step forward is like building a home: one brick at a time. Are you going to stop half way and give up on completing your house? Or are you going to focus on the final goal of moving into a new home? Once you start building, you can only go upwards; regardless of how long it takes, you will eventually reach the point where your roof will be up.

For years, I made the mistake of disregarding the little steps. I thought that acquiring a skill, like playing piano for example, is more of a decision as to *when* to start rather than creating a habit of consistently taking the little steps. The possibility that I could achieve such a goal by taking even minuscule steps never entered my mind. To begin with, I was already discouraged by the "bigness" of the idea. I was under the impression that something like that had to be started "at the right time" (whatever that meant); that I would have to plan it thoroughly, give it a clear "starting date"— like turning it into my New Year resolution. I was more concerned about starting at the perfect time, then starting and following through consistently. Every beginning of the year I made very clear plans about my desired goals— in fact, you should've seen my yearly planners! I always took the time to write down my long lists of things to do for the upcoming year. Things like, "Learn how to play the piano", "Study music theory", "Start writing my next book", and "Record my first Christmas album". I always purchased my yearly planner months before the New Year and chose it very carefully, convinced this little book held the answer to my life's success.

However, after more than 15 years of buying fancy yearly planners and entrusting them with all of my dreams, I was still in a place in which none of my goals were accomplished. Fifteen years later, and I was still not able to play piano whatsoever (in my defense, I did buy an electric one), I still didn't start on my music theory rudiments (of course I bought the manuals), I had only written the title of my new book, and didn't record 1 Christmas song. Fifteen years of living my life without doing some of the things I always knew would make me a happier person. Even though I was driven and clear in what I wanted to achieve, the results were never what I had hoped. And as years went by, I became increasingly baffled by that.

I was yet to learn that making the choice and starting the process were only part of the answer. I didn't know the rest of the story, the being steadfast stage. I didn't know that temporarily going off course (something we may call "failing") means absolutely nothing in front of persistence and patience; that no matter how small my steps were, as long as I was steadfast, I would eventually create the habit. And that habit is what would make it happen for me in the long run— not the decision I initially made, but the habit. The habit, which I was supposed to nourish day in and day out despite of how many times I didn't felt like doing it.

There is a good reason as to why many New Year's resolutions fall flat on their faces soon after they're started. Sometimes we fall into the I-gotta-stick-to-my-plan-no-matter-what-'cause-if-I-don't-the-whole-thing-is-ruined trap. Life kicks in and you happen to deviate from your original plan a little bit; you had a birthday party and ate a cupcake, missed the morning run, had that extra glass of wine. You have to stop making it sound like it's the end of the world if you happen to have gaps in your consistency. It's the consistency *over a long period of time* that counts, not the little hiccups along the way. These little stops truly don't mean anything if you just pick yourself up and continue where you left off.

How many times have you made a plan, only to automatically decide that you failed the first time you missed a day or two? According to my colorful yearly planner, I would start on the day I said that I would, but something would come up and I'd miss a day of practice. Then I would be all wired up and disappointed because "I failed to stick to the plan". The next day something I could've easily said "No" to would come up, but "...since I missed my last practice and the entire plan is ruined anyways", I would say "Yes" to it, and miss yet another day. Then I would consider the whole thing a big fail and get overwhelmed by an avalanche of negative emotions, such as guilt and lack of trust in myself.

First of all, it's not the end of the world if you miss a day. It's not the end of the world if you miss 2, or 3, or even 4 days. What's important is that you do it consistently over a long period of time. Even if that means 1 day a week instead of 5 as you originally planned. As long as you consistently do it, over a long period of time— such as one year— IT WILL ADD UP. For example, if you went jogging for 1 hour once a week (instead of 3 to 5 times per week as you presumably planned), at the end of the year it would add up to 52 hours of jogging. Let's assume that you weigh 160 pounds— you can burn 581 calories in one hour when jogging 5 mph, which at the end of the year adds up to roughly 30,212 burned calories, or the equivalent of 8.6 pounds of fat. I'm not implying that you should only do 1 hour of jogging a week. The purpose of this example is only to highlight that even if for some reason you don't follow your initial program and do it less, it doesn't mean that it won't work. The key is to—

simply— do it. Maybe you won't get to the desired results in the time frame you originally expected, nevertheless, you will get results. Also, by continuing to do so you give the body the chance to create the habit, and that's what counts more than anything. Now that the habit is formed, it will turn around and support you.

I can only imagine where my piano playing skills would've been, had I practiced ONE day a week for the 20+ years that I had been longing to learn. When I thought of THAT, is when it hit me. My next move? I started waking up every morning 30 minutes earlier than usual to study my piano and music theory. Thirty minutes— no more than that. Then something interesting happened. Because I didn't make it such a big deal, "Ooo, this is big, it's my NEW YEAR RESOLUTION!", I was more relaxed when it came to having to stick to the plan. As a result, and to my total astonishment, I barely missed any practice times. Only months later, I passed my first Royal Conservatoire Music Theory exam and received First Class with Honors. I was in my early forties.

The idea is to focus on one thing at a time. There is something magical that happens when you take one idea alone and give it your best shot. By putting all your focus and energy into it, it kind of has no choice but to come to reality. Even if, let's say, you do have the mental and physical stamina to take on more than one project at once, I would still not recommend it. Working a little bit on many different things will take longer to accomplish. As a result, you might run out of patience because you don't see results sooner with any of them. When you put all your focus and energy into one clear goal, you can make it happen faster. Then you can move onto the next thing. Make small changes; if you never worked out before, don't start with a 5 day a week training routine *and* completely change your diet at the same time. You could get overwhelmed and rebound to your old habits.

I'd say the first step is to THROW OUT YOUR SCALE. You don't need to keep count of every ounce you lost because you know that once you do the right thing you can only go forward. If anything, your clothes will let you know if you're moving in the right direction. However, I wouldn't count much on that either, especially in the beginning when the body weight tends to fluctuate before it can fully adjust to the new eating and exercising habits. Once you have the right habits, once you keep it simple and give the body what it needs, you will get to the image you want without having to keep score of how much weight you lose each day. Just do the right thing and leave the rest to your body. You can start, for example, with creating the habit of walking more. You can make some small changes in your diet at the same time, such as eliminating soft drinks. Stay with that for a while, let your body get accustomed to the change— have patience. When you feel it became second nature, implement a couple more changes, like choosing the right kind of dairy products— avoid the ones with complicated ingredient lists, avoid words such as *homogenized, modified, processed, added sugars, artificial sweeteners, colors*, and so on (I'll discuss this more in the Nutrition chapter). Also, don't complicate yourself by getting these foods only for you. Get your entire family involved in eating right as well, help them create some positive habits of their own.

You choose whatever changes you feel comfortable making. Introduce a new habit as your last new habit becomes stronger, but don't do it all at once. And make sure you keep that desire alive, but don't let it ruin your patience. Impatience is the biggest trap and the reason why so many people fail to achieve their goals. Give it a year, give it 2 years if need be. I know it sounds like a long time but time passes anyways. Two years from now you could be looking back at the same you, or you could be looking back at a much different you. Arm yourself with patience and know that you can do it, simply because it's all up to you and nobody else— you are in full charge. In the beginning you might not feel like that's the case, but as you overcome the negative habit and strengthen the positive one, you will feel more and more in control. And as your new good habit becomes automatic, the path to your goal will become clearer: a matured positive habit is like a powerful spotlight highlighting the sureness of your destination, so now the distance and the time it takes to reach your goal become irrelevant— *because now you know you are going to get there.*

Don't disregard the little steps and you will be living a different story altogether. In doing so, now you open the door through which God can come and work His magic. Prepare to be amazed now because God's steps are not little. He can, in an instant, turn a life-long struggle into a beautiful conclusion that will bring you all the happiness you've been imagining, plus interest— He can do that. God can make it all happen. But start valuing the power of your own little steps, decide to take them already and follow through. As I said before, although your steps are small, they are extremely powerful. That's because as soon as you take the first one and follow up with the next, then the next and the next, you are doing much more than creating a life-promoting habit.

Now you're showing God that you are ready to accept His universal leap.

Part Two:

the Practice

Chapter 4

NUTRITION

HOW *NOT* TO DIET

My grandmother Urania (who I call *mamutza*) lived out in the country, in a very small village in Romania. She had lots of chickens, goats, ducks, pigs, and grew all her fruit and vegetables. Her way of living, like most farmers back in Romania at the time, was very simple: no electricity, gas, or running water. She used petroleum lamps for light, a wood-burning stove for cooking and heat in the winter, an outdoor water well for water, and a small outhouse for a bathroom. Even though such living conditions might sound harsh to some, I personally couldn't wait at the end of every school year to leave my city apartment and spend my summers at mamutza's, barefoot.

I absolutely adored my mamutza. She truly loved her farm life, and at the same time she had the attitude of a gentle queen. Even though life threw at her heartbreaking curbs, she never made an issue out of her struggles. Instead, she quietly took circumstances as they were, moving through life with dignity and complete lack of self-pity.

Mamutza had a natural ability to see things differently; when talking to her, she never gave an answer or remark I would normally get from someone else. She always put her own twist on things, making one think there could be other possibilities residing outside the box most of us live in. I was very bubbly one day, telling her how I could not wait to start my first year at university, when she put an interesting twist on the idea of higher education: *"I don't know about all that school... You have to be careful. It can turn you stupid instead"*.

Mamutza was very adamant about what she was feeding her family, which was very unusual at the time. I was a teenager when a new product called *Vegeta* (a powdered vegetable stock) hit the shelves in the city. Very excited about this new culinary wonder, my mother brought a pack to mamutza. *"What's this?"* mamutza asked, clearly not impressed by the colorful packaging. *"It makes your food taste better"* my mother answered. *"Why, what's wrong with my food?! And what's inside?"*, mamutza continued questioning. *"...Lots of dried vegetables and some other things that give food flavor"* my mother answered slightly confused, probably wondering why she was getting interrogated all of a sudden. *"Well, I can't see what's inside so I'm not going to use it"* mamutza concluded.

SHE COULD NOT SEE WHAT'S INSIDE. Although for some reason that stuck with me, I never really got it until years later...

As I mentioned earlier, weeks after I arrived to Canada I started feeling inexplicably sick. Headaches, acne, PMS, brain fog, irritability, increased anxiety, heart palpitations, eczema on my knees and elbows, digestive problems, were some of the issues I was suddenly faced with. Something even more frustrating than going through all that, was that none of the doctors I knew at the time could give me an answer as to why I was so sick all of a sudden, or why my symptoms magically subsided every time I would travel back to Europe. For more than 4 years I persistently tried to find an answer, which I finally got when I began studying fitness at Seneca College in Toronto...

As soon as I started school, I knew it was the best decision I made in a long time. I loved every single course in the program however, Nutrition was one course that surprised me the most and drastically changed things in my little universe. What I learned in the next few months made me very passionate about this subject. My nutrition teacher came to class one day with her hands filled with different product labels. It seemed odd, to say the least, that she would strip boxed foods of their colored labels. But I went along with it. She started talking about how reading labels was the most important thing you can do for your health, aside from being physically active. I was confused— what do you mean "read labels"?! The only part of the label I used to read was the price! But as it turns out, the ingredient list holds the secret to our health. That was something very new to me— newer than when I saw the no-touch faucet for the first time once I arrived in Canada. (You should've seen the expression on my face while looking to find the knob of the faucet in a fancy public bathroom. I even looked under the sink!)

Back to my Nutrition teacher, apparently, things we eat can make us sick. Many of the ailments people suffer from nowadays are caused by foods. Or *things added* to the foods we eat, to be more precise. In order to prolong shelf life, many of the foods on the market today are excessively filled with food additives. As a result, they cause people to gain toxic fat deposits and can trigger hundreds of illnesses, as already proven by scientific research.

I was staggered to learn that foods can contain more than just natural enzymes, naturally occurring sugar, or fats. Where I grew up there was one kind of everything:

one kind of bread, one kind of oil, one kind of sugar, one kind of yogurt, one kind of milk... you get my point. I don't remember ever having a choice of anything. If we wanted butter, we went to the store and got the only butter there was. I know this might sound terrible, but I'm starting to think that was best, since all foods were in their most basic, truly natural form. I noticed that the vast array of choices available today— the interminable variations of the same product— create sort of an anxiety in people. Like the constant sprouting on the market of new versions of yogurt: "The new, fat-free, sugar free, lactose free yogurt that improves your digestion". How can people *buy* that? In Romania, where I grew up drinking raw dairy regularly, it was a known fact that once the milk was boiled, it's pretty much dead. Boiling (a form of pasteurization), strips it of its natural enzymes, which are actually the ones that AID in the digestion process. After going through all the processing procedures in the big factories, I don't think that that "new and improved" yogurt has anything left from its original shape, form, or composition.

I don't think it is yogurt anymore, period!

And how can anybody improve something that was perfect to begin with?! You milk a cow and get perfect milk, filled with enzymes and other amazing nutrients your body recognizes and digests easily. It's impossible to turn that into a better milk because perfect is perfect. It's like saying, "I don't think nature did a good job on this oak tree. Let me genetically modify it in a lab and make it better".

Mind you, I think they do that already...

Going back to my nutrition teacher, as she continued, I got my big "AHA" moment. As I was growing up, I never heard of children fighting obesity, having allergies, asthma or diabetes. I had never heard the words "breast" and "cancer" put together in the same sentence, PMS, or menopause. When I moved to North America, my eardrums were suddenly inundated with all these strange words, with the most common one being "allergies". In Romania we used the word "allergy" only when referring to a person we didn't like— we would say "I'm allergic to that person", meaning "I don't like that person". When I went to see my family doctor in Toronto for the first time and she asked if I had any allergies, I was a bit perplexed that a doctor would actually ask me if there was someone I didn't like!

I never gave one thought to the foods I ate; didn't think the apple I was eating in Canada is different in any way from the one I ate when growing up in Romania. As a matter of fact, when I first went in a grocery store in Toronto, I was spastically happy (remember my adoration for food). I had never seen such a diversity of fresh fruit and vegetables put together under one roof in my entire life! And so many jarred goods lined up on the long shelves, like mayonnaise and cheese spreads that (strangely) didn't need to be refrigerated!

Then it was the fast food restaurants, which I had never seen before. A few times per week I used to pay homage to these giants, amazed at how they never failed to feed people with incredible promptness and out of this world constancy of taste. At the same time, the all-you-can-eat restaurants were one of my absolute favorite places to park in for about half a day. The small kitchen counter in my Toronto apartment was always overstocked with wholesale size boxes of chocolate, sugary processed cereals, and instant dried soups that magically swell up to "real" soup once covered with hot water.

I was mesmerized by all this newness and easiness of eating!

Now, my nutrition teacher tells me to READ THE LABELS!

When I got back to my apartment that day, I ran like a bullet into the kitchen and, to my total stupefaction, there was not one product I had that didn't have some ingredients I couldn't read!

I had no idea how I could sort all this new information in my head and have it make sense to me, so that I can successfully implement it in my daily routine. Then I remembered what mamutza had said when my mother handed her the new flavor-enhancing product: *"I can't see what's inside so I'm not going to use it"*. I realized I had to de-focus from the confusing labels, reach for mamutza's truth deep within, bring it out, and find a way to mesh it with my new reality.

When I go to the grocery store now, I keep her in mind and ask myself, "Would my mamutza approve of this product? Would she use it in her kitchen? DO I KNOW WHAT'S INSIDE?" I soon discovered that the selection of truly natural foods available in grocery stores was pretty limited. And as a result, the amount of foods I was buying reduced drastically (and so did my monthly food expenses). It wasn't easy to break the seemingly comforting habit of buying previously prepared foods, but I kept at it like a programmed robot. Only weeks later, I woke up one morning and didn't feel as tired. To my total astonishment, my symptoms started disappearing.

We all want to make better decisions for our families, for ourselves. On the other hand, it's very easy to get caught up in this incredible vortex of diet trends and fads circling around us at such high speed, it truly can make one lethargic. Most of the time, our eating habits are the result of decisions we make based on the information we are given— and that, we are given plenty of nowadays. In their quest to grab a bigger slice of our stomachs, some of these companies work so hard at trying to outdo one another, to the point where their information becomes downright antagonist to each other: eggs yolks are bad for your cholesterol vs. the fats in egg yolk is good for you; don't eat butter, it has saturated fats vs. butter is good for your brain; eat kale, it's the most nutrient dense food vs. raw kale affects your thyroid; red meat is bad for you vs. red meat is a great source of B vitamins, Iron and Zinc, etc... It became a daunting task— to say the least— to find the right answer in this colossal mess of information. The answer to "WHAT IS BEST TO EAT?" doesn't come around easily anymore. The simple act of eating turned from being one of the most natural and joyful things to do, to a legitimate source of anxiety and stress.

As a result, too many of us give up and choose a frozen dinner instead.

My mamutza's seed of simplicity is what I will be trying to reveal to you here. It is exactly that: SIMPLE. I'm telling you right now, it doesn't have to be hard and it actually is not. You just have to be willing to put a bit of initial effort into it, just until you start eliminating your unsupportive habits. Getting rid of habits you've had for a long time (even decades for some) is not easy— I'm not going to claim that it is. But once you remember your reward, once you clarify your positive outcome, hold on to it like you would hold on to a branch while dangling down into a dark, bottomless valley— like it's a matter of life and death. Put your entire focus on your reward, and it will carry you to the other side.

Very important, surround yourself with people who approve of your decision and are genuinely supportive. Don't give a second thought to the peanut gallery trying to drag you down. Look at them as people who probably have their own challenges, their own unwanted habits. Although it doesn't happen that often anymore, I find it amusing when someone decides to ridicule Giuseppe and me for our ongoing enthusiasm in taking proactive steps towards better health: "What, you want to live forever?" (Which to tell you bluntly, out of all the negative remarks I had to hear over the years, I crown this as the least intelligent one.) Obviously, how long one lives cannot be predetermined. What you *can* predetermine though, is to be as disease-free as possible, have the energy to run and play with your kids, have the drive to explore new possibilities, maybe even do things you never thought you would have the drive to do, regardless of age.

When you take charge and create better habits, your entire life— including of those around you— can and will change for the better.

My passion for wellbeing didn't stop once I graduated college. As the subject of healthy eating is continuously being tackled by highly regarded scientists, doctors and nutritionists, I've always been turning to these experts to keep myself aware of the latest research. These are passionate people who are dedicated to finding the truth about how the human body works. After years of research, they got to the point where they can firmly say, "It's scientifically proven". So I can't possibly bring you a different answer because the right answer has been numerously relayed to you already. I'm here to offer nothing new.

Only a different perspective: my mamutza's.

You might wonder, where do habits fall into all this? They do, and very much so. Everything that involves eating starts with a habit— from the section of the grocery store you shop mostly in, to the kind of foods you choose to eat on a regular basis, to the quantity you eat at one meal, to the restaurants you choose, to how often or how rarely you cook at home... These are all habits. If you don't like the taste of raw broccoli, plain yogurt, or kefir, it's not because these foods taste bad but because your taste buds have been consistently flooded with processed foods— which created a habit of preferring them instead. Once you understand that almost everything we do is habitual— including the foods we eat— you'll realize there is no such thing as "I don't like kefir" but simply "I'm not *used to* eating kefir". This puts *you* in charge and not your taste buds. In this scenario, you own the power of decision and are able to control your taste buds as to what foods to approve of. Via your habits, you can get yourself to the point of actually enjoying foods you previously considered tasteless.

There is another point I'd like to make here. Giuseppe likes to bring this up occasionally, and I happen to think it's a pretty valid idea. He calls it the "lasagna paradigm" (of course the man loves his lasagna!).

...Imagine you're hungry. In your mind's eyes you see dancing before you a fresh, out of the oven, steaming lasagna, overflowing with gooey mozzarella cheese. You want that lasagna so much, you would do almost anything to sink your teeth into it. But... there is no lasagna available in that moment (I don't know, maybe you married a Romanian girl or something...). Anyway, let's say there is absolutely no way you could get that lasagna in that moment. What you do have available however, is a boring piece of chicken breast and some broccoli. You have no choice, so you eat it. Now you're fed. Now you're not hungry anymore.

Do you think you would still crave the lasagna?

Hunger doesn't care what you eat. Once you ate, you're not hungry anymore. And once you're not hungry anymore, you don't crave the food that's bad for you (not that lasagna is bad for you because it's not, provided it's made with ingredients free of food additives and you eat it in moderation). My point here, in order to be successful at creating a habit of eating healthy, you have to be mindful in the moment in which you make the decision as to what kind of food to reach for. Are you going to reach for the store-bought sweet, filled with modified milk ingredients, food coloring and high fructose corn syrup? Or are you going to reach for a couple of dates and a few nuts? If you're mindful and reach for one of the second choices, you will most likely not crave the unhealthy treat anymore. And now you made a life-promoting choice.

Use the common sense of simplicity. Think "mamutza" simple: EAT FOODS THAT ARE IN THEIR ORIGINAL NATURE-INTENDED SHAPE, FORM, and COLOR— I like to call them *simple* foods. Simple foods contain no additives, are not grown with pesticides (for fruits and veggies), hormones or antibiotics (for meats), and are non-GMO.

Complicated foods, on the other hand, contain much of everything I mentioned before, and sometimes more. Aside from being used to enhance the flavor of our foods, additives are also intended to lengthen their shelf life, prolong freshness, and enhance appearance. With a bit of initial due diligence, (like simply turning the product over and reading the ingredient list) it can be easy to pinpoint which foods are complicated and which ones are simple. Avoid foods that are in a form they don't naturally come in— like that spreadable cheese in a jar found in the no-need-for-refrigeration section of your supermarket. You feel like something sweet? Bake some cookies from scratch. It's good for you and makes nice memories with your kids.

There are very few packaged foods I personally get and if I do, I always read the ingredients first. If it's cereal, I only choose the ones with the least ingredients as possible, such as brown rice (or corn) and sea salt. If it's potato chips I want, I select the ones that are baked and have short ingredient lists, such as potatoes, sea salt, and oil.

As I mentioned before, I had a long-term sugar addiction. It's been many years since I beat it, something I achieved by eliminating all complicated foods from my diet. It's scientifically proven that regular consumption of processed foods, especially the ones sweetened with high fructose corn syrup, create an unnatural sugar dependency. I don't avoid foods that are considered fattening by many, such as breads, pastas, or fats (like butter for example). However, I do pay attention that they are simple— they don't contain additives— and I eat them in moderation. I don't mind organic brown sugar or raw sugar— but I do mind processed white sugar, fructose, artificial sweeteners, and high fructose corn syrup. I don't mind a fresh white flour baguette made with non-GMO or organic unbleached flour, water, salt, and yeast— but I do mind that unnaturally soft, white, sliced bread, which contains more tongue twisting ingredients than what's in your medicine cabinet. I don't even mind a little extra good quality Himalayan or sea salts— but I do mind table salt.

Table salt may be contaminated with sand and glass, two abrasive elements that cause small tears in the arteries. Some people would argue the fact that regular table salt has iodine added, an important nutrient needed for proper thyroid function, while some of the healthier choices don't contain iodine. Although that's true, I prefer to get my intake of iodine in a supplement form, rather than eating regular table salt and having to worry about high cholesterol, clogged arteries, and possibly cardiovascular disease.

Up to this day, I still follow my mamutza's philosophy of simplicity. But did I dread having to read all labels in the store in the beginning? Of course I did. I was furious! But I also knew that that was only temporary. It really wasn't long before it all became second nature. Now, I simply head to the small healthy foods area of my grocery store and automatically get the familiar products I know are good for my family. When I first learned from my nutrition teacher in 1999 to read labels, there was a limited amount of simple foods in our grocery stores. Today, there is a wide variety of healthy foods; a movement, which fortunately grows bigger every year.

It would be nice, however, if some of the all time North American favorite sweets were made without harmful additives. Giuseppe was particularly disappointed to learn about the effects of regular consumption of food additives on the body. There are store bought treats he used to have as a child, which now he stopped getting. Occasionally, he passes by the isle stocked up with his childhood favorite treat and reads the list of ingredients, hoping that the manufacturer changed them for better. Most of the times I see him put it down with a frustrated expression on his face. Other times though, he sneaks it into the grocery cart and enjoys it with his expresso the next day. Which is fine. The point here is not to be radical. As long as a large percentage of the time you make healthy choices— as long as you give the body a chance to cleanse by eating simple foods— the few times that you do eat something with additives are not enough to accumulate in the body to the point where it can cause issues.

Since 2001 I've been feeding my family what I think is best: foods which are as close to their original state as possible. My husband Giuseppe and I bake often. We don't deprive our 15-year old daughter— or us for that matter— of the joy a chocolate chip cookie can give. But we bake it with quality organic ingredients, found in their simplest form. And yes, we spend less money in the process as well.

At the same time, we are not extremists. If we're invited for holidays, a birthday party or a wedding, we are going to eat what we're served. We don't starve ourselves because the food is not healthy. What's important is that most of the time we eat simple foods— and that makes the whole difference.

THE REASON WE GAIN WEIGHT

"Is this fattening?" is one question I've been asked numerously and still being asked up to this day. "This" standing for a wide range of foods such as butter, oil, pasta, bread, sushi, whipped cream, avocado, full-fat yogurt, etc. I say this as lovingly as I possibly can, for all of you out there who keep asking this question: no foods are fattening unless they are complicated (aka, processed foods). Aside from cases where there is an existing medical condition that contributes to weight gain (such as an underactive thyroid), we gain weight because we eat complicated foods, we overeat, and/or we don't combine protein, fats and carbs at each meal.

Eating complicated foods

Simple foods are recognized by your body. As a result, it breaks them down easily and positively utilizes their nutrients— yes, even if it's butter. Complicated foods on the other hand, contain foreign substances (such as food additives), which are not recognized by your body; therefore, it cannot properly break them down (low-fat, fat-free, and diet beverages fall in this category as well). Once invaded by these toxins the body goes into a "safe" mode, a state in which it locks them into fat cells and stores them away— usually in the hips, thighs, waist... we know the "problem" areas very well. Creating fat cells to store harmful toxins (as opposed to allowing them to roam freely) is the body's way of protecting you from illness. Day after day of ingesting complicated foods, our bodies work relentlessly to keep us alive, by creating fat cells that hold prisoners these harmful chemicals— the more we eat, the more fat cells the body will create to store these toxins. Hence why we get heavier and heavier during a time when low-fat/fat-free/diet products are still popular.

Let's take the fat-free yogurt as an example. Yes, it has less calories than the full-fat version (125 calories, as opposed to 150 calories). However, your body will end up storing much of the 125 calories because of the artificial food ingredients that are added to improve its taste. In the case of the full-fat yogurt, your body will store none or close to none of the 150 calories, provided you don't overeat.

Another example is honey and white sugar. One teaspoon of sugar has roughly 16 calories, and 1 teaspoon of honey has about 22 calories. Both honey and white sugar contain glucose and fructose. Glucose is what gives an immediate increase in energy levels. Fructose, on the other hand, converts into energy at a slower rate, resulting in increased energy for longer periods. This natural process is being facilitated in honey because its glucose and fructose are separate. In comparison, the glucose and fructose in white sugar are bonded together. This makes it hard for the body to positively utilize them and ends up storing them as fat.

In conclusion, even though honey has more calories, those calories are positively utilized by your body in the form of increased energy levels. As opposed to the fewer calories in white sugar, which the body is not able to fully utilize and ends up storing.

Overeating

This is pretty straight-forward and simple: based on your average daily activities and bodily functions, if your body needs 2,100 calories to maintain its weight but you ingest 2,500 calories, over time you will gain weight— even if it's simple foods you're mostly eating. Logically, if you do both— eat complicated foods *and* overeat— you will gain even more weight.

The question is now, how do you know when you crossed the line over to the "I overate" territory? Yes, you could count your calories but I believe there are simpler, yet valid ways to keep overeating at bay. The following are 3 practical measures that can help one overcome a possible overeating habit, something I personally do:

- Put on your plate only the amount of food you know you should be eating, and STICK TO THAT ONLY
- Eat slowly
- Chew longer

Put on your plate only the amount of food you know you should be eating, and stick to that only— I cannot stress enough how important this is. Make it a rule that you don't go for seconds. Should you still be inclined to do so, here is a trick I learned from a client I used to train in the gym: before you start eating, put on a belt— not too tight that it makes you uncomfortable, and not too loose that it hangs down. Notice how your tummy fills up as you eat. As soon as you feel the belt becoming slightly tight, stop eating.

You could also experiment with this: once you're finished eating what's on your plate put the fork down. Wait 20 minutes, then notice if you're still hungry. It takes roughly 15 to 20 minutes for the brain to receive the message that the stomach is full. When you wait, you allow this process to take place and most likely won't feel like eating more than you need to. By doing this consistently, you create a habit of listening to your body and not overload it.

Eat slowly— at one point or another, all of us experience intense hunger and may eat super fast when food becomes available. Although we might not always realize, inhaling food is a habit. But if instead you remember that your prefrontal cortex is there to assist in making better choices, you will create a habit of taking control over your hunger and eat slower as a result. Relaxing in front of a meal and enjoying every bite is a habit that can be easily developed. Just like any other habits, it will take some time to become automatic. But once it does, you will discover the true joy even the simplest meal can offer.

Chew your bites longer— your stomach will thank you for sending down smaller food particles that are already partially digested; this occurs when the food has a chance to mingle with the saliva in your mouth long

155

enough, which also results in better digestion and less chances of being bloated after dinner.

Not combining protein, fats and carbs at each meal

Aside from not overeating this is probably one of the best eating habits you can create for yourself, particularly if you're looking to lose weight. When at each meal you combine lean protein, healthy fats and complex carbohydrates, your insulin levels become steadier and your body will not store fat (again, provided you don't overeat). As a result, you will also have stable energy throughout the day. According to Dr. Barry Sears, author of New York Times bestseller *A Week in the Zone*, *"My research showed that if you were able to keep insulin levels within a certain zone— not too high and not too low— you could dramatically improve your health and prevent a wide range of diseases. What's more, you could also make your body start using fat for energy, thus allowing you to lose excess body fat without feeling hungry!"*

Protein:

Lean meats, fish, all beans, eggs, tofu, edamame, hemp seeds, even spirulina, are sources of great protein. Create a habit when you're hungry to **always look for protein first.** A quick and easy way to get your protein intake when you're in a hurry is to have hard boiled eggs in your fridge at all times. Another great way to get your adequate protein intake is to find a good, additives-free protein powder and have a protein shake instead of a meal. Whey protein (non-isolate) from cow or goat milk that came from grass-fed animals (or better yet, organically raised) is my favorite. B if you're lactose intolerant, hemp or soy protein powders work great, provided they have as little ingredients as possible.

Fats:

You probably heard "Eat fat to lose fat". According to Dr. Barry Sears, when insulin levels are not steady (which happens when we don't combine protein, fats and carbs at one meal), the body ends up storing more fat. Eating good fats in moderation will not make you gain weight. Your body will break it down easily and your tummy will feel satisfied. Skip the saturated fats (such as the ones found in fatty meats and chicken skin), and choose the monounsaturated and polyunsaturated ones. Best sources of healthy fats are cold pressed oils (olive, sesame, avocado, peanut), fish, nuts and seeds (also in the form of nut butters), avocados.

Something else to take into consideration is that eliminating healthy fat from our diet can cause various symptoms such as dry skin, mental fatigue and poor body temperature regulation. It affects hormone synthesis, bone health, the reproductive system and most importantly, it affects the nervous systems and the brain. According to Dr. David Perlmutter, eating the right amount of fats helps keep dementia at bay: *"Welcome fat back to the table. It's good for the heart, brain, immune system and just about every aspect of human physiology you consider. And as it specifically relates to dementia, new research clearly shows us that individuals eating more of the 'dreaded' fat actually have a substantial risk reduction for becoming demented while those with diets favoring carbohydrates the risk for dementia dramatically increased."*

Carbohydrates:

There are 2 main types of carbohydrates: complex and simple. Complex carbs are not processed and are rich in fiber. Some examples of complex carbs include whole fruit, vegetables, legumes and whole grains (brown rice, pastas and breads made with whole flours). These types of carbs are loaded with fiber, which is a main ingredient in keeping your insulin levels steady.

Refined carbs on the other hand, include anything made with white, refined flour (pastas, bread, pastries, white rice), fruit juices, and beverages sweetened with sugar. They will cause spikes and dips in your blood sugar levels, which is one of the reasons for weight gain.

LISTEN TO YOUR BODY

One day, farmer Vasile isn't feeling well and goes to see the doctor. After an extensive check up, the doctor gives him the bad news: "Farmer Vasile, you have cancer in stage four." Farmer Vasile is shocked to hear that and asks the doctor "Is there anything I should eat?" "Nothing will make it go away" the doctor crushes his hope. "Just go home and eat whatever you want because you have two more weeks to live."

Farmer Vasile goes home and decides that since he's going to die soon anyway, he might as well indulge in his favorites: red wine and steak.

Six months later the doctor's office door opens wide and a glowing farmer Vasile enters. "Doctor, I feel great! I think the cancer went away!" Astonished, the doctor asks with a stutter, "...You gotta tell me what you did!" To which farmer Vasile answers cheerfully, "I drank red wine and ate steak every day!" The doctor pulls out his notebook and writes down what he now believes to be the breakthrough cure for this type of cancer: "Steak and red wine".

The next day, accountant Petru goes to see the doctor. He, too, suffers of the same type of cancer, with months to live. "Don't despair", the doctor rushes to comfort accountant Petru. "I have the cure for you. Eat steak and drink red wine every day. Farmer Vasile did that, and he was cured."

Accountant Vasile goes home and does just that, but 3 days later, he suddenly dies.

Confused, the doctor picks up his note book and writes his conclusion: "Red wine and steak: good for farmers, very bad for accountants."

This is a popular joke my father used to tell when I was growing up. However, I always had a feeling that it was more than just a funny joke.

Could there be a reason behind why certain diets work well for some people and not so well for others? And could this reason be at the heart of the infamous *"Results may vary"*?

Eat Right 4 Your Blood Type Diet by Dr. Peter J. D'Adamo says "yes". After explaining the origin of blood types, Dr. D'Adamo underlines how foods that are normally regarded as healthy can be toxic for certain blood types. By "toxic" he doesn't mean *complicated* foods. In fact, foods that are extremely well regarded like chicken, sesame seeds, lentils, and avocado make the list. For example, I have blood type B and chicken with polenta (one of the staple foods in Romanian cuisine, Moldavia to be exact), may cause serious health issues with long-term consumption. Same with lentils, avocado, coconut oil, sesame seeds, and corn— organic or not, GMO or non-GMO, these foods are particularly toxic for people with blood type B. As soon as I eliminated these foods from my diet, I felt a definite positive change in some of the issues I was experiencing for a long time, one of them being chronic low blood pressure.

As I mentioned in the introduction, I'm not a hired spokesperson for anybody and this diet is no exception. I choose to speak about it simply because it made a positive change in my life. But if this idea doesn't appeal to you, the next best thing you could do is listen to your body. If a certain food you're eating is not good for you, your body will let you know; you just have to pay attention. Once you're done eating, are you feeling energized or sluggish? What does your tummy tell you? Does it feel settled or bloated? Do you have a bellyache or heartburn?

I'd like to tell you a personal experience I had with one of the best regarded food remedies there is: chicken soup. As I mentioned previously, I used to suffer of low blood pressure. I don't mean to sound like a spoiled brat, I know many people battle high blood pressure. However, low blood pressure can be problematic as well, especially when it reaches dangerous low levels. Once I had to be admitted in the emergency because my blood pressure reached such lows, I was constantly fainting for about 6 hours.

I did take my doctor's advice to drink more coffee and have a glass of red wine at dinner. But that only worked temporarily and I needed something that can actually *fix* the issue.

Then I went to see a naturopath who explained to me that most people suffer from leaky gut at one level or another (due to regular consumption of soy, dairy, and gluten), which can be a legitimate cause of many different symptoms, from fatigue, arthritis, nutritional deficiencies, gas, constipation, bloating, poor immune system, to even depression, anxiety, and autoimmune diseases. He recommended that I fix the leaky gut and see if it would resolve my chronic low blood pressure.

After the consultation, I had a meeting with a client of mine who happens to be a strong advocate of healthy living, and the subject of leaky gut came into the conversation. She then proceeded to tell me that a few years before she suffered from leaky gut, which she fixed by eating chicken soup only. She recommended that for 3 days in a row I eat organic chicken soup for breakfast, lunch, and dinner.

That advice kind of made sense to me; boiling chicken with bones for a long period of time pulls out certain enzymes from the bone marrow, which is what gives the chicken soup its healing properties. It inhibits infection caused by cold and flu viruses and fights inflammation due to the anti-inflammatory amino acids, such as argentine.

So before I went to the health food store to get the product my naturopathic doctor recommended, I thought why not give it a shot with chicken soup first? We all know the curative benefits of chicken soup— hey, they even wrote books titled that way, so it must be good!

The first day I ate my organic chicken soup I did not feel any better. As a matter of fact, my abdomen felt somehow *heavy*. But I thought nothing of it.

The second day I ate my organic chicken soup I DEFINITELY did not feel better. The only word that kept popping in my head when looking down at my abdomen was "angry". That's how I felt my tummy was— angry.

The third day, I was ready to sit at my table in the morning and have yet another bowl of organic chicken soup, when I felt so sick to my stomach, I thought I was going to throw up. I couldn't even look at the soup, let alone eat it. I thought to myself, "You're not supposed to feel sick from chicken soup! What's going on?"

The body is very smart. We should at least be as smart and listen to it once in a while. After my 3-day chicken soup adventure, I still continued eating this well-regarded protein and felt sick every single time. But I never made the connection between my not feeling well and eating chicken. I had such a strong belief that chicken is good for everybody— my "chicken-is-the-best" neural pathways were so strong— that not even for a second did it occur to me to consider otherwise.

Only months later, I learned from *Eat Right 4 Your Blood Type* that chicken is purely toxic for my blood type. Why I had to see it written in a book before I trusted the signals of my own body, is beyond me. As soon as I eliminated the chicken and the rest of the foods that were toxic to my blood type from my diet, my blood pressure normalized and it's been stable ever since.

You are unique. Nobody in this entire universe was, is, or will ever be identical to you. Therefore, your nutritional needs are unique. Some foods might be healing for some and not so healing for you— hence my chicken soup experience. Don't get stuck into a template and brush off physical discomfort, just because the experts are saying it's the best program/diet ever invented. Take the advice but at the same time pay attention to your body's signals. Learn what works best for *you*, not what works for the "majority".

You don't want to be part of the group of people who get the shorter end of the stick of "RESULTS MAY VARY".

FOOD ADDITIVES
— Anything But Simple —

The foods we eat today are not like they used to be 30, 20, or even 10 years ago. That salami, those biscuits, that bread, milk, or yogurt you see today, even though they might look the same, they are not. To my Italian mother-in-law, the veal cutlets she gets today are no different whatsoever from the veal cutlets she used to get 50 years ago when she moved to Canada— simply because it is impossible to see a difference. How could she *"see"* the antibiotics and/or hormones the calf was given, or the pesticides and GMOs in its feed? The more you try to explain how detrimental eating that meat could be, the more she resists by rhetorically asking what I believe to be an incredibly valid question: "If it's so bad, why would they sell it?!"

I clearly remember when I first started learning about the effects of food additives on our bodies from my Nutrition teacher... I was so incredibly confused! As if an alien world opened its doors and let an avalanche of questions pour in, with the main one being "Why would anyone create something that hurts people?" Then again, we didn't know smoking was going to be the cause of such radical diseases until much later. Now we're learning more and more about the negative effects of lab created substances added to our foods. Wait and see, eventually we'll get to the point where everybody will take seriously the negative effects of EMF and Wi-Fi on our bodies...

You might, too, wonder why these unnatural ingredients that have already been linked to numerous diseases ended up in our food in the first place. The answer is, because they have been designated as *"Generally Recognized As Safe"* (GRAS) by certain experts. I could understand where the experts are coming from; in the beginning nobody thought smoking could have such deep negative consequences. Only years later, when there was an increase in lung and heart related diseases, did researchers look closer into the long-term effects of smoking cigarettes. It seems like it was yesterday that people were smoking inside their houses, cars and restaurants, a behavior considered illegal today.

Same with food additives; until proven unsafe by scientific studies, nobody suspected that Monosodium Glutamate (MSG) was going to be a cause in susceptible individuals of severe chest and/or facial pressure, overall burning sensations in the digestive system, and sometimes a heart attack-like feeling. Nobody really knew that with prolonged ingestion it could precipitate severe migraine/headaches in some adults, cause asthma, eye damage, fatigue, depression, disorientation, numbness, heart arrhythmia and palpitations, brain damage and/or worsening of Alzheimer's and Parkinson's disease. Nobody suspected that it was going to be one of the causes in our obesity epidemic, as well as a link with epilepsy-type "shudder" attacks in predisposed children. Nobody suspected that the detrimental effects of ingesting

MSG would be so extensive, that entire nations— entire continents, such as Europe and Australia— would ultimately have it banned.

The amount of information available on food additives is so unbelievably extensive, it made it quite difficult for me to put it in a context that's comprehensive, yet concise— reason being, food additives are anything but simple. It might seem that my telling you about it defeats the simplicity I promised in the beginning; however, something I noticed over the years is that most people eat foods tainted with additives simply because they genuinely have no idea the extent these foods could affect their health— they genuinely have no idea that the negative effects that may occur due to long-term ingestion of these toxins oscillate between mild, all the way to disastrous in some cases. I've seen it over and over, where once people are given the information, they decide to make a change. Maybe we don't need to fill our minds with all the horrifying details. But I believe we need to at least have the knowledge that food additives exist, so that we can make an informed decision as to what to feed our kids.

When it comes to understanding the full extent to which food additives may affect one's health, I personally didn't need much convincing. As I mentioned earlier, I felt firsthand how these toxins could burden the body years ago, when I moved to North America and became exposed to them for the first time. As this happened during a time when the research was not so easily accessible (before we had at our fingertips the vastness of the World Wide Web, as Optimus Prime would say ☺), it was extremely rarely suspected— if at all— that something inside our foods could be a legitimate cause of many of our ailments. For many years researchers, doctors, and scientists around the world have been relentlessly studying these toxins and their long-term effects on our bodies, and are continuously releasing papers and reports that show staggering results. I consider this information so paramount to humanity's well-being, I truly think it should be taught in elementary school.

The problem today is that we're caught in a vicious circle; we got too used to someone else preparing our meals: we became conditioned to think that only foods in colorful packages and perfectly looking fruit and veggies are worthy of our hard-worked money. We got conditioned, just like with everything else, to favor what *looks good*. Apples are not naturally blemish free and covered with a layer of what many of us assume it is "wax" (which in many instances is Diphenylamine, a harmful food additive meant to create a glossy sheen and keep fruit fresh for longer). Pickles are not really supposed to be bright green in color, and those kid's cereals do not naturally come in all the colors of the rainbow. In them there are additives that create an artificial shell, much like Photoshop turns a skin from blemished to glowing with a spectacular golden hue— when in reality it's not. Did you know that out of the nearly 4,000 different additives currently in use, more than 3600 are used exclusively for cosmetic reasons? Did you know that some food manufacturers actually add preservatives to pickles, when in actuality the very act of pickling *is* preserving? Yes, pickling preserves perishable foods for months, making them last longer. The brine (water and salt) preserves the cucumbers in the most natural, healthy, pro-body way. However, because the color of the pickles tends to naturally fade during the preservation process, some food manufacturers add preservatives to stop their color from fading. Why do they do that? Allow me to answer with another question: how many people do you think would choose pickles that have a poopy, fainted green color?

It ultimately comes down to what people choose. If we all choose the bright green pickles with tongue-twisting ingredient lists over the truly natural version, that is exactly what food manufacturers are going to keep manufacturing: bright green pickles with tongue-twisting ingredient lists.

Some would argue that additives are present in foods in such minute quantities, that they are harmless. This is almost tolerable when we consider that the human body can detoxify some additives; however, most additives have been shown in different studies to be both mutagenic and carcinogenic, which means the human body is not able to detoxify easily. When these additives are consumed on a regular basis— in even minimal doses— it will eventually result in a toxic load on the body. And toxicity leads to many dreading diseases, including cancer.

Another point is that even though a product may contain micro quantities of additives, in the end it adds up to a large quantity when most of the foods one consumes contain additives.

All that being said, you should not have to give up your favorite dishes, stop eating foods that you love. But you can improve on the ingredients you habitually cook with If your family is used to having veal cutlets once a week, switch to organic or grass-fed veal and use GMO-free breadcrumbs. Fry them in a little bit of grape seed oil (which has a high smoking point and won't turn toxic), or bake them and sprinkle olive oil at the end to add some moisture and healthy fats. If your mother made macaroni and cheese once a week when you were a child and you're continuing the tradition, make sure you use the healthy versions of the same ingredients over the processed kinds. Making these changes will get your family off food additives gradually, and that is extremely important considering food additives are addictive—something that shocked me when I first learned about.

When consumed on a regular basis, food additives affect the taste buds on your tongue, making them crave that particular food over and over. As a result, they create an unnatural, almost obsessive behavior— it gets you addicted to that particular taste, similar to an addiction created via regular use of drugs or alcohol. Then when you do venture and try to eat simple foods, you'll find them bland, tasteless. It's this addictive element created by food additives that makes it hard to switch from processed foods to simple foods.

You might or might not be surprised to hear that processed organic foods can also contain additives. I had a rather disappointing experience with a certain brand of organic bouillon cubes. I personally don't use store bought bouillon in my cooking, but many people I know do. Unfortunately, most of them use the more affordable versions filled with many food additives, one of them being the infamous monosodium glutamate (MSG). For the longest time I recommended the organic version— you know, the one that says "no MSG, no GMO" in bold letters on the front of the package. One day I was outraged to find out that some of their ingredients— like *yeast extract* and *natural flavor*— actually ARE or may CONTAIN MSG.

Just because a label says, *"Organic, no MSG, no GMO'*, does not guarantee it's a healthy product.

Are your taste buds dumbed down, desensitized by additives? If they are, then now they have to be trained to like the taste of simple foods. Which is not an easy task,

I'm not going to sugar coat it. However, having the whole picture on food additives (as researched by numerous scientists around the world), can make it easier to make a change and stick with it. Apples, carrots, eggs, full fat yogurt and so on, don't create dependency. I believe the very fact that additives create an addictive behavior should be enough information for anyone to want to initiate a change.

Excitotoxins

I've been asked by many people, if I were to give ONE advice as to what to eliminate from their diet first and foremost, what would it be? Would it be bread? Would it be pasta or sweets? Would it be red meat?

My answer came very easily: none of that.

What you should eliminate from your diet TODAY is EXCITOTOXINS. You can probably imagine their surprise at the sound of that. The truth is, excitotoxins are the real bad guys— the kind you want to snap your fingers and make them instantly disappear from the face of the earth.

Excitotoxins are food additives created with genetically modified bacteria which stimulate taste receptors on the tongue. They are basically *"...chemicals added to foods to make them 'tastier'"* explains Dr. Cathie Lippman, founder of the Lippman Center for Optimal Health. *"Excitotoxins cause a brain cell to become very excited and your neurons basically fire spastically until they finally burn out."* Lippman explains.

Here is another explanation given by Dr. Theresa Ramsey, a highly regarded naturopathic physician, lifestyle expert and author: *"These substances excite neurons so aggressively that the nerve impulses fire rapidly and repeatedly until they become exhausted. These neurons become excited to death and hence have received the name 'excitotoxins'."*

It is speculated that 90 percent of migraine headaches are linked to consumption of excitotoxins, due to their overstimulating nerve cells until they are damaged or dead. This puts migraines and headaches first on the long list of health issues researchers found to be caused by regular consumption of excitotoxins. Even small amounts of excitotoxins will unleash the symptoms in someone who suffers with regular migraines.

Excitotoxins also cause high levels of free radicals leading to cell death. They were found to change brain chemistry leading to an array of serious conditions, such as strokes, brain injury, brain tumors, Alzheimer's, Parkinson's and Lou Gehrig's diseases, meningitis, neurological Lyme disease, encephalitis, schizophrenia, and have been directly linked with aggressive and violent behavior.

Russell Blaylock, Neuroscientist, author, and former professor at the University of Mississippi Medical Center, wrote in his 2007 Blaylock Wellness Report: *"Newer studies have shown that feeding MSG to animals not only dramatically increases the free radicals and lipid peroxidation products in the walls of their arteries, the increase lasted for what would be the equivalent of decades in humans."* Blaylock continues to say *"...we now know that the excitotoxic process plays a major role in many life-threatening maladies."*

Unfortunately, the effects of excitotoxins do not stop at the brain and nervous system. According to Dr. Theresa Ramsey, they also cause irritable bowel syndrome (IBS), fibromyalgia, chronic fatigue syndrome, and overburden the immune system which has to work overtime in order to protect the vital organs from these toxins.

Excitotoxins do not discriminate; they affect everyone who ingests them regularly. However, kids can be affected at much deeper levels. When infants are given foods that contain excitotoxins, the effects might not be seen until later, when damages might already be present in the form of disorders in the endocrine, learning, or emotional levels. Also, due to their highly addictive properties, once kids are used to eating them at an early age, it will be much harder to make changes later in life. Dr. Russell Blaylock states in his book *Excitotoxins: The Taste That kills:* "Hundreds of *millions of infants and young children are at great risk and their parents are not even aware of it. It is my opinion, after reviewing an enormous amount of medical and research literature, that MSG, aspartame and other excitotoxin additives poise an enormous hazard to our health and to the developing and normal functioning brain. To continue to add enormous amounts of excitotoxins to our food is unconscionable and will lead to suffering and ruined lives for generations to come."*

So what exactly are these excitotoxins?

The main excitotoxins are **Glutamate** and **Aspartate**. Generally, you find Glutamate in savory processed foods such as canned soups and broths, while Aspartate is mostly added to soft drinks and sweet foods.

Glutamate

Here is Dr. Ramsey's descriptive explanation of how Glutamate, MSG in particular, can cause addiction: *"... excitotoxins are used in high levels in all processed foods (fast foods are processed)* as flavor-enhancers, and because of their makeup are also highly addictive, remember, "bet you can't eat just one?" MSG for example is so flavorful that it imparts a fifth level of taste in addition to the four basic tastes of sweet, sour, salty and bitter, it also gives us a taste called 'umami' which is Japanese for savory. The taste creates an addictive quality along with the 'excitement' that these chemicals cause in our bodies. With these chemicals in our foods, it truly is impossible to eat just one and manufacturers count on it so you'll keep buying it and keep coming back to the drive-thru as often as possible as you unknowingly continue to crave these 'exciting' chemicals."

When it comes to Glutamate, the main ingredient written on the packaging of processed foods containing this excitotoxin is Monosodium Glutamate (MSG). However, today Glutamate is, or is part of, many other food ingredients that sound nothing like it.

Keep in mind also that aside from the ingredients that are listed on the packages, some of the processed foods contain hidden amounts of Glutamate that are not required to be listed on the label, partially because they are considered to be present in *"small quantities"*.

The following is a list of food ingredients present in processed foods which, according to experts, may contain Glutamate or in which glutamate may be created during processing: wheat gluten, autolyzed yeast, milk protein casein, calcium caseinate, gelatin, gelatin protein, cysteine, glutamic acid, monopotassium glutamate, sodium caseinate, texture protein, yeast extract, yeast food, aspartic acid, yeast nutrient, hydrolyzed soy, wheat, pea, whey and corn protein, flavors, flavorings (no, they are not the same), seasonings, natural flavors and flavorings, soy sauce, soy protein isolate, soy protein, bouillon, stock, broth, malt flavoring, malt extract, barley malt, carrageen, maltodextrin, protease, corn starch, anything protein fortified, anything enzyme modified, anything ultra-pasteurized.

It may be safe to assume that any processed foods— organic and non-organic— may contain Glutamate.

Aspartate

When it comes to the excitotoxin Aspartate, the story is similar to that of Glutamate. Aspartate is a food additive categorized as a Sweetener, and is widely used by the soft drink and sweet food industry. Aspartame and Saccharin, both containing Aspartate, are on the list of powerful excitotoxins. Aspartame can be found in over 6,000 products (usually sugar-free or diet products) such as: instant breakfasts, cereals, yogurt, milk drinks, gelatin desserts, juice beverages, topping mixes, cocoa mixes, coffee beverages, shake mixes, soft drinks, sugar-free chewing gum, tabletop sweeteners, tea and coffee beverages, instant teas and coffees, wine coolers, breath mints, as well as in some over the counter medicines and supplements.

Like Glutamate, ingesting artificial sweeteners on a regular basis can change the way you taste food. They can make you avoid highly nutritious foods in favor of artificially flavored ones that have less nutritional value. In an interview conducted by Holly Strawbridge (former Editor at Harvard Health), Dr. David Ludwig, an obesity and weight-loss specialist at Harvard-affiliated Boston Children's Hospital explains *"Non-nutritive sweeteners are far more potent than table sugar and high-fructose corn syrup. A miniscule amount produces a sweet taste comparable to that of sugar, without comparable calories. Overstimulation of sugar receptors from frequent use of these hyper-intense sweeteners may limit tolerance for more complex tastes. That means people who routinely use artificial sweeteners may start to find less intensely sweet foods, such as fruit, less appealing and unsweet foods, such as vegetables, downright unpalatable."*

As there is a plethora of scientific research showing the undeniable negative effects of Aspartame, some food manufacturers started replacing it with newer artificial sweeteners. The problem is, due to the fact that some of these ingredients are still new, there's not enough scientific research done showing their possible impacts on our health. Aspartate may be found in many artificial sweeteners, such as acesulfame potassium, aspartame, corn syrup, cyclamate, erythritol, fructose, glycerol, glycyrrhizin, hydrogenated starch hydrolysate (HSH), high fructose corn syrup (HFCS), isomalt, lactitol, maltitol, mannitol, neotame, polydextrose, saccharin, sorbitol, Sucralose, and more.

Weight gain is one issue related to consumption of artificially sweetened drinks and foods. In an article published online in 2012 titled *Fueling the Obesity Epidemic? Artificially Sweetened Beverage Use and Long-term Weight Gain*, the San Antonio Heart Study documented weight change in men and women over an 8-year period, and offers evidence that there was a double risk of obesity in those drinking diet beverages compared with those who did not drink them. In a study involving adolescents, intake of artificially sweetened beverages was associated with increased body fat percentage. *"These findings raise the question whether artificial sweeteners use might be fueling—rather than fighting—our escalating obesity epidemic."* the article concludes.

The American Heart Association (AHA) and American Diabetes Association (ADA) have given an alert in regards to the use of artificial sweeteners in their Journal of the American Heart Association. After conducting several studies in order to identify the association between diet soft drink sweeteners and chronic disease, such as heart and kidney disease, they concluded that people consuming 2 servings of diet soft drinks per day were at an increased risk of these particular chronic diseases.

Studies show that excess fructose can lead to higher triglycerides, a risk factor for heart disease, and decreased insulin sensitivity, a precursor to diabetes. *"Fructose is mostly responsible for the increasing risk for metabolic syndrome – obesity, hypertension, poor cholesterol parameters, kidney disease, fatty liver, type II diabetes, accelerated aging, memory loss",* Dr. Theresa Ramsey underlines. *"Labels that read – 'no sugar added' means that no 'table sugar' is added BUT companies can put in fruit juice with these labels – which have more fructose in it than HFCS. Obesity in 1975 occurred in 15% of the American population. Now, 34 years later obesity rates are > 50% of the population. Americans ate less than ½ pound of fructose per person in 1980. Now, Americans eat 50 pounds of fructose per person per year. The greater intake of fructose has been linked to the dramatic increase in obesity; 2 out of 3 people in the U.S."* Recent studies from the University of Oxford reveal that high fructose corn syrup *"can increase the risk of Type 2 diabetes, which is one of the most common causes of death in the world today."*

When it comes to sucrose, excessive consumption of it has been directly associated with a high incidence of antisocial and criminal behavior. Stephen Schoenthaler and his team from California State University conducted several studies among thousands of incarcerated juvenile offenders, and found a link between high sucrose and junk food intake and the occurrence of disruptive, antisocial behavior. *"After replacing sugary drinks and junk food snacks with fruit juices and nutritious snacks with 276 incarcerated offenders, informal disciplinary actions were lowered 48%, when contrasting the twelve months before, and after nutritional revision. Assault and battery was lowered 82%, theft 77%, horseplay 65% and refusal-to-obey-an-order 55%. The consumption of sucrose/additive-rich foods was not only seen to worsen the behavior of young offenders, but when given to children diagnosed as hyperactive, these foods seemed greatly to increase their restless and destructive behavior. Excessive refined carbohydrate consumption can also lead to a disordered carbohydrate metabolism. Reactive hypoglycemia has also been associated with diverse personality and psychiatric disorders, such as neuroses, panic attacks, agoraphobia and schizophrenic episodes."*

Aside from excitotoxins, there are other food additives that should be avoided like preservatives (benzoates, sulphites, nitrates), color additives (food coloring), flavors and flavor enhancers. Fortunately, most of them are found in processed foods, which means that once you ditch processed foods for the reason of avoiding excitotoxins, you also eliminate other food additives that may be in them.

GENETICALLY MODIFIED FOODS

Genetic Modification (or Genetic Engineering) is the process of manipulating an organism's genome (its DNA) by changing the genetic makeup of cells including transferring of genes from a foreign organism, for the purpose of creating a new or "improved" organism.

Genetically Modified Organism (GMO) is an organism whose genes have been altered through genetic engineering techniques, so that the final product contains genes that are not normally or naturally found in the organism's original form.

Genetically Modified foods (GM foods) are foods that were produced from Genetically Modified Organisms (GMO) by means of Genetic Modification.

Why should we avoid GM foods? Here is a fact: as of 2015, more than two thirds of European countries banned GM foods because have been shown to cause harm to humans and animals. The environment is also affected by the practice of genetic modification because GM crops are heavily sprayed with herbicides that seep through the soil, polluting our earth and water. The herbicide Roundup used on GM crops is also found by experts to immobilize nutrients, which means you could be eating greens all day, but the nutrients will not be physiologically available for your body. Dr. Don Huber, one of the world's leading experts in GM foods underlines: *"You may have the mineral (in the plant), but if it's chelated with glyphosate, it's not going to be available physiologically for you to use, so you're just eating a piece of gravel."*

Ideally, all GM foods should be avoided. However, if that's not feasible, here are 11 foods that would be best to be avoided in a GM form: corn, wheat, soy, sugar, aspartame, papaya, canola, dairy, zucchini, and yellow squash.

So how do we stay away from harmful additives? By simplifying what we eat. Eliminate all processed foods from your kitchen. We arrived at a point in our civilization where in order to restore our energy levels, attain optimal weight, balance ourselves emotionally and mentally— in order to restore our wellbeing— we have no choice but to be radical. Remove ALL foods that contain additives.

Start by first eliminating the additives that can do the most damage: the excitotoxins. Whether you choose to do it the cold turkey way or implement small changes as you go, in the end the goal should be one: to get your family off the excitotoxins as soon as you possibly can. The simplest way to do that is by going back to the basics: bypass the processed food isles all together. Choose foods that are in their original shape and form, and are non-GMO. Remember what I said earlier, stick to the predictable simple foods list.

Once you do that, there's not going to be much left to change in your diet, unless you decide to go organic. And switching to organic foods is a much easier process (by swapping the regular broccoli with the organic version, for example).

When it comes to creating a habit of eating and enjoying simple foods, you need to have patience and an open mind, be willing to put in the time and effort to make the changes. This could be a delicate matter because, as I mentioned earlier, additives create an addiction in the taste buds. Switching to eating simple foods could be especially hard on kids. Dr. Ramsay approaches this subject eloquently: *"Many parents ask, 'how do I wean the fast foods and bagged snacks from my children?' The most important thing is to be gentle, go slowly and get them involved with understanding how their body responds to different foods. Kids know when they have headaches or they are tired or wired when bedtime comes. The more you sit and educate and take time with them and offer other healthy foods they will slowly come around. Our taste buds change over every 3 weeks – BUT – the neurotoxic effect that excitotoxins have on our brains take 6-12 weeks to break that 'addiction'. It is time, patience and keeping many options for children to keep trying over and over again. You can go cold turkey and endure a higher level of pain for a short period – but this is more typically much more successful for adults. Mindfulness and love are the backbones to success in changing eating patterns in all people."*

I'm often asked by parents what snacks are better to give their kids. The first thing I tell them is to try to avoid the already prepared snacks, simply because so far, I haven't found a kind that doesn't contain some sort of additives. It is safer to stick to fruits, raw veggies like celery and carrots, a piece of cheese that contains no tongue twisting ingredients, a home-made cookie with oats and nuts, or my version of fruit yogurt (plain yogurt with jam). Some nuts and dried fruit bars may be ok however, I read their ingredients to make sure they don't contain anything else that's not supposed to be in there.

Depending on their age, kids don't always comprehend the idea that ingesting these toxins long-term could affect their development and impact their future as a result— but *you* know that. You also know that, although in the beginning it might be a struggle to have your kids break old habits and implement new positive ones, the end result will be undeniably worth your time and effort. I believe having compassion as a parent is not giving into what our children cry for, letting them have that store bought "treat" filled with dubious ingredients. Having compassion as a parent is making an effort to guide our children toward making healthier eating habits; it's making time to bake for them *real* treats— the kind that are not only tasty, but are filled with genuine nutrients that can nourish their bodies. Our kids could have more energy, better focus, and experience less bothersome illnesses. Even more importantly, they'll start collecting immeasurable interest in their health bank, something they'll very much appreciate later in life.

ORGANIC FOODS

The USDA National Organic Program requires that *"Organic food is produced by farmers who emphasize the use of renewable resources and the conservation of soil and water to enhance environmental quality for future generations. Organic meat, poultry, eggs, and dairy products come from animals that are given no antibiotics or growth hormones. Organic food is produced without using most conventional pesticides; fertilizers made with synthetic ingredients or sewage sludge; bioengineering; or ionizing radiation."*

It's wonderful that scientists keep us up to date on the effects of complicated foods on our bodies. By being well informed, we know what to stay away from when grocery shopping.

However, I think we arrived at a stage where we focus a bit too much on what *not* to eat; I think we put too bright of a spotlight on how all food additives can affect our health. At this point in time, the scale of our attention is heavily tilted toward what to stay away from. This is a real problem because there are more unhealthy foods than actual simple foods on the market today. To put it simply, the list of complicated foods became exponentially longer than the list of simple foods. And since we usually spend more time talking about what's unhealthy, it's only normal to get exceedingly overwhelmed and not be sure of what to eat anymore. The matter is becoming increasingly worse, as the already long ingredient lists keep getting longer and more tongue twisting.

Therefore, I came to the conclusion that it would make more sense to keep in mind the shorter list (the simple foods list), which is more or less the same today as it was during our grandparents' time— I don't think nature will come up with a brand new vegetable any time soon. The beauty is that once you know this list, you know it for life. It's simple and predictable. The research has been done and thankfully will continue to progress, which is great because it helps us make informed choices. But let's do our part also and support the farmers and manufacturers that have genuine care for our planet and the people living on it, by sticking to the simple food list when shopping for groceries.

If you and your family consume fast foods on a regular basis, switching to simple foods would be a big step in the right direction; like replacing frozen fries with home made ones. Eating organic, on the other hand, is taking your diet to another level, and I believe is the ideal scenario.

I know people who think of organic foods as some sort of fad, a "Silly, rich people's phase" I was even told. "Organic foods are too expensive, I can't afford it", is another one. What's interesting is that most people who said that to me are either smokers, eat out regularly, or their form of entertainment during weekends is shopping for clothes they don't really need.

No judging, just sayin'...

For the sake of the argument though, let's say you're a non-smoker, you mostly cook at home, and you're happy with your existing wardrobe. In that case no worries, I still have a few more arguments:

1. **We do not need half the foods most of us habitually get.** Sometimes, while waiting in line at the grocery store, I can't help but notice the kind of products the person before me unloads on the rolling band, and I have to admit I get a bit irritated. I get irritated to see that most of the unhealthy foods are for kids: flavored yogurt, pop, fruit juice concentrates, highly processed cookies and cereals, snack bars sweetened with high fructose corn syrup, frozen fries, frozen pizzas and chicken nuggets, ice-cream and other wanna-be milk dessert products containing modified milk ingredients, among other things. "But my kids won't eat anything else" is the common excuse I hear repeatedly. My question is, what if salmon with broccoli and rice was the only food available on the planet? And the answer never fails in coming quickly: "They won't eat it." Yes, maybe for the time being. But what if they have nothing else to eat the entire day? Will they actually let themselves starve? I can assure you that if they're hungry, they will eventually eat anything you put on their plate.

A few years ago, my sister-in-law came over for a visit with her 3-year old. At one point, my little niece asked for one of those flavored yogurts packaged in small colorful plastic containers. I don't have a habit of getting that particular yogurt, but I figured I could maybe "trick" her into eating my daughter's own version of it: organic, non-homogenized, full-fat plain yogurt, to which she adds a layer of strawberry jam. I go open my fridge, and to my total embarrassment I realized I was out of yogurt! Now I found myself in a pickle but didn't want to give up. So instead of yogurt I used kefir. I honestly didn't think she would eat it, as kefir is more of an acquired taste. But to my total stupefaction my little niece ate it all, then *she asked for more!*

I can assure you that switching from those small fruit yogurt containers to making your own (by purchasing the bigger containers of yogurt and jam), is not only far healthier, but more affordable as well.

So many kids eat unhealthy nowadays (and parents pay the price quite literally) because we are not willing to put up with tantrums, or because we *assume* there is going to be a tantrum. I'm not trying to make anyone feel guilty; as parents— especially mothers— we have plenty of valid excuses to do so. Juggling between work, family and extra curricular activities, became a job on its own. But the bottom line is, if we want our kids to be healthy, if we don't want to spend unnecessary time at the doctor's office, then it would make sense to put in the effort and help them create better eating habits.

2. **Organic foods are more perishable, so big grocery stores usually put them on sale a few days before their expiration time.** When it comes to meats, get a bunch when on sale and freeze them as soon as you get home. In the long run, what you'll pay for organic meats is the same (if not less) than what you pay for non-organic versions.

3. **Something else to keep in mind is bulk foods.** There are wholesale chains that carry organic foods at affordable prices. It's not a secret to my family and friends that I love shopping at Costco. I know where everything is now, so it only takes me 30 minutes to be in and out.

However, once in a while I do venture outside the familiar aisles in search for new food products. In many occasions, my face suddenly lights up at the sight of yet another product available in "mamutza approved form"— like organic, unpasteurized honey for example. When I saw it at Costco for the first time, I thought I reached heaven! As soon as its golden hues hit my retina, I grabbed two of them, and before putting them in my cart I gave them a big, long hug. Sure my husband didn't want to be associated with me in that moment (I could tell by the way he disappeared all of a sudden). By the time we got to the car I had already texted everyone I knew: "1 liter of organic, unpasteurized honey at Costco for $7.99! ☺ ☺ ☺"

4. **Lastly, we should consider being more economical and not waste food.** There are 2 aspects of being wasteful: eating too much, and throwing food in the garbage.

Eating more than your body actually needs is just as bad as throwing food in the garbage. Not only you're wasting money by eating what you don't actually need, but your body has to work twice as hard to digest the extra food, *and* you could be gaining unwanted weight. In conclusion, overeating is a waste of food, money, and health.

In regards to throwing food in the garbage, maybe it's the Romanian in me who grew up during the times when most foods were rationed. But the bottom line is, being more mindful of how much you cook so food doesn't end up in the garbage adds up in the end, regardless of whether it is organic or non-organic foods.

A SIMPLE PLAN

My idea of simple is thinking about it in terms of food groups. I took the liberty of playing around a bit with the categories in the widely known food group pyramid. You'll find that some of my recommendations are real simple: non-GMO (or organic), or avoid all together. My philosophy is this: if a food doesn't have the potential of nourishing your body, if it doesn't at least maintain your health let alone improve it, it's simply not worth it.

That being said, I'm not suggesting you suddenly turn into a robot. As long as most of the time you eat simple foods, the occasional bought burger, donut, or your mother-in-law's lasagna can't hurt you. My personal simple foods-complicated foods ratio is roughly 95%: 5%, but only because I choose to. I believe eating simple foods even half the time, would be an improvement for some.

Water

Water... What a simple idea it used to be! If someone said 30 or so years ago that in the near future we would be drinking water from harmful plastic bottles that sit for who knows how long in the hot sun or freezing temperatures, turning what's supposed to be life-giving into what researchers found as a link to many diseases (i.e. asthma, attention-deficit disorders, breast cancer, obesity, type 2 diabetes, neurodevelopmental issues, low IQ, autism, male fertility issues, altered hormone levels, heart problems, increase risk of cancer, stomach pain, vomiting, diarrhea, stomach ulcers, retinal bleeding, spontaneous abortion, etc.)— AND PAY MONEY FOR IT— we would've shouted "Get out of here you crazy, that can NEVER happen!"

Well, we let it happen.

Phthalates, a group of chemicals that make plastics flexible and softer, are used in almost everything— from water bottles, food packaging and household cleaners, to fragrances, personal care products, and cosmetics. The studies are there already, backing up all these claims. In one of its publications, *Environmental Health Perspectives* notes: *"Phthalates (known as plastics) are the number one toxin in the human body. Phthalates are so potent that if a mother is drinking out of plastic water bottles while she's pregnant, she can be programming her unborn child for adult diabetes, poor brain and nerve function, breast cancer, to name just a few."*

Another concern with plastic water bottles is the BPA content (Bisphenol A). BPA is also present in various foods containers, sports equipment, CDs, and DVDs; epoxy resins containing BPA are used to line the inside of various food and beverage cans. A study from the University of Florida published in the *U.S. National Library of Medicine* has found that the plastic used in water and soda bottles can release antimony and bisphenol A (BPA) if it's exposed to heat over a long period of time. BPA came more into the spotlight a few years back, when scientists discovered that some plastic containers leach BPA into their contents. Even the bottles that come with the "BPA free" claim attached to them may not exactly BPA free.

Lena Ma and her team at the University of Florida also studied the effects of heat on water placed in plastic bottles that are BPA-free, and the team detected trace levels of BPA in the samples. *"In theory, the plastic should not contain BPA,"* Ma says, *"One explanation is that during the manufacturing process, especially when recycled plastics are used, trace amounts of BPA may be present. It's an impurity."*

In the online journal *Fertility and Sterility*, senior research scientist Dr. De-Kun Li shows that BPA may change men's sex hormone levels. *"BPA is similar to the female hormone estrogen, meaning that it could have effects on the human body. The effect of BPA on men may be more immediate and easier to detect than the effect on women, because men have very low levels of estrogen to begin with"*, Dr. Li said.

Another study from China suggests that exposure to this chemical may lower testosterone levels in men. According to the study, men who are exposed to BPA from working in a chemical plant for at least six months have lower levels of testosterone in their blood, compared to those who work in a tap water factory.

All that being said, let's move beyond the plastic bottle issue and look at the ever-increasing types of water available on the market today. How do we know which one is best to drink? That becomes a very important question because according to experts we are made of 60% to 75% water and need to drink a lot of it in order to stay healthy. You don't necessarily need water to stay hydrated; you could be drinking 6+ cups of broth or freshly squeezed juice daily and you'd be just fine. But that's not realistic, so we have to rely on other sources of hydration and water is the handiest one.

But there is a catch... Even if you drink 6 to 8 glasses of water a day, it doesn't necessarily mean you're hydrated; most of the time the water we drink settles in between the cells and turns into extracellular fluid, or what we know as *water retention*. In order for the body to be hydrated, the water has to reach inside the cells. *"A person's vitality is affected by how well his or her body gets water into and out of cells"* says Elson Haas, an integrated-medicine physician California and the author of *Staying Healthy with Nutrition*. One of the main issues people complain about when drinking bottled water (including my husband and I) is that it tends to "sit" in the stomach. When this happens, it could be a good sign that the water you're drinking is not really hydrating you.

Another quality water should have, aside from hydrating your cells, is the right pH level. In other words, it shouldn't be too alkaline or too acidic. When you drink water with the right pH level, as well as free of contaminants, your cells will become hydrated. This translates into maintaining a healthy body weight, having glowing skin, better circulation, proper food digestion and absorption of nutrients. It also helps decrease muscle and joint inflammation and supports your body to detoxify naturally. So which water can do all that?

Tap water— is out of the question; depending on where you live, it can be contaminated with arsenic, aluminum, fluoride, chlorine, and prescription and over the counter drugs.

Alkaline water— produced with one of those alkaline water machines available on the market today is, according to some experts, too alkaline for the body. Although in the first couple of weeks of use it can help detoxify, drinking alkaline water long-term invites various health issues, especially for people who already battle with digestive problems. Alkaline water reduces the acid needed to break down and absorb food, which could lead to diminished good bacteria in the gut. This can further facilitate the development of other digestive problems, such as ulcers and parasitic infection.

Distilled water— is considered by some too acidic. Research shows that although over a short period of time it, too, can help detoxify, drinking it long-term will draw minerals right out of your body and possibly create health problems.

Water filter— Some experts say that the Reverse Osmosis Filter, Ion Exchange Filter, Granular Carbon and Carbon Block Filters are some of the best choices because they remove different contaminants in tap water. Having one of these filters in your home is healthier and more economical than bottled water; it keeps your family away from harmful plastics and helps our planet in the process as well.

Natural spring water— aside from getting a good filter for your house, you can also look for a natural spring water in your area. When you drink spring water, you need not to worry whether it's too alkaline or too acidic. Depending on where the spring water is coming from, it can contain various amounts of healthy minerals, like Sulfur for example. Sulfur is an essential life mineral found in muscles, skin, and bones. It's needed for insulin production, helps with detoxification at cellular level and relieves pain, among other things.

There is a wonderful website called *FindASpring.com*, which gives the locations of various potable water springs in North America, as well as around the world. You'd be surprised to learn how many springs exist around the world and the high number of people who take advantage of this gift of nature.

Water in a nutshell:

- Avoid water in plastic containers— spare your body and the environment of harmful plastics
- Install a water filter in your home
- Find a source of spring water in your area

Vegetables and Fruit

Choose non-GMO or organic when possible

When it comes to fruits and vegetables, my choice is simple: organic. By eating organic, you bypass harmful pesticides and genetic modification.

Non-GMO fruits and veggies are the next best thing; I personally wouldn't choose them over organic as they most likely contain pesticides and herbicides, but it certainly is a better choice over the genetically modified versions.

Save money by getting fewer fresh veggies and fruits at one time, and avoid throwing food in the garbage. Alternate veggies so you don't limit your intake of vitamins and minerals.

Get fruit and veggies in season & freeze them

The abundance of in-season fruits and veggies produced locally comes with the benefit of being less pricey and tasting better. We tend to think that most fruits and veggies grow in the summer only but that's not the case. As a matter of fact, many of the fruit and vegetables we think grow in the summer actually taste better when harvested in the fall, such as artichokes, arugula, beets, broccoli, rapini, figs, eggplant, edamame, kale, carrots, celery, chard, cauliflower, garlic, grapes, squash, apples, endives, and mushrooms. While citrus, pomegranates, bananas, kiwis, winter squash, watercress, turnips, potatoes, radishes, turnips, leeks, rhubarb, parsnips, are seasonal to winter.

Take advantage of the lower prices and nutrient-rich produce by purchasing your fruit and veggies in bulk and freezing them. Freezing locks in nutrients and flavor, while giving you the benefit of having supplies for the rest of the year.

Ferment vegetables

Before refrigerators, fermentation used to be the way people preserved food to make it last longer. Fermenting is not only a safe way to make foods available all year round, but its tremendous health benefits are now recognized by esteemed doctors and researchers. Having a balance between the good and bad bacteria in the gut results in physical, emotional, and mental well-being. And since it's a natural probiotic, the living bacteria in fermented foods also helps improve your immune system. Approximately 80 percent of the immune system is found in the gut. Every time you ingest probiotics, you increase your good bacteria, resulting in a stronger immune system.

Another positive aspect is that the living bacteria in fermented vegetables make them more digestible and help break down other foods in the digestive tract. Aside from their unparallel health benefits, yet another upside of fermented vegetables is that they require no cooking; they can be enjoyed as a side dish with almost any meal, and only a small amount is enough to get their benefits.

One of the epidemics of our century is unnatural weight gain, which in many cases leads to obesity. Obesity may also occur as a result of unhealthy gut bacteria due to eating foods that lack in probiotics. The effects of probiotics in our bodies are so positively extensive, top neurologists in North America such as David Perlmutter recommend introducing them in your diet as both, a supplement and in the form of foods.

Last but not least, fermented vegetables are highly detoxifying. The probiotics existent in these foods assist the body in detoxifying from many toxins, as well as heavy metals.

Already prepared fermented vegetables free of additives can now be found in grocery stores, which is great. But if you want to make your own (and also save money in the process), you'll be happy to hear that fermenting is quite easy to do; all you need is vegetables, water, sea salt, and jars. Almost any vegetables can be fermented, from carrots, cauliflower, red and white cabbage, string beans, parsnip, celery root, green tomatoes, beets, ginger, garlic, watermelon, turnips, eggplant, cucumbers, onions, and squash, even watermelons. In Romania, where I grew up in the region of Moldavia, fermenting small whole watermelons is as normal as fermenting cabbage, and it actually tastes surprisingly good.

Grow some of your own

As much as having a vegetable garden would be ideal, you don't necessarily need a backyard to reap the benefits of an enzyme-rich leafy vegetable or a handful of fresh parsley, rosemary, or basil. There are quite a few ingenious innovations out there, such as compact towers, which make growing vegetables in your apartment or house easy.

If you do have a backyard but don't want to make a designated area for a vegetable garden, as long as you make sure you have decent quality soil, you can plant vegetables anywhere on your property. Aside from planting them in pots, you can use the space in between your flowerbeds, by the fence, and around the base of your trees. You can even take it to the next level and throw in some red worms to increase the amount of air and water that gets into the soil. Worms are often called "angels of the earth" or "free farm help" because they eat what we don't need (like leaves and grass) and leave behind castings that are the best kind of fertilizer for your vegetables.

There is an indescribable feeling of gratification that comes from spending an hour in your garden, taking care of those little plants; seeing a little seed materializing into a beautiful fruit filled with life-giving enzymes and nutrients. I applaud individuals such as John Kohler of *Growing Your Greens*, whose enthusiasm and commitment to educating people in growing their own fruit and vegetables, is truly admirable.

Plant an organic or non-GMO fruit tree

One of the very first things I noticed when I moved to Canada was this frenzy of planting regular trees in the backyards, front yards, on the side of the road, along sidewalks, in parks, even on the edge of already treed areas. The town plants a (non-fruit) tree in front of each newly built house, and that's great. I get it, we help the environment.

But how about helping the environment *and* feeding people at the same time? How about letting nature plant its own maple trees where it decides, and us plant fruit trees instead? Can you imagine a street filled with apple, pear, cherry, apricot, or plum trees from which kids and adults in the neighborhood could just pick? I can, and let me tell you, there is a freedom in that that cannot be explained. Nature knows how to take care of everything in a way that it doesn't hurt anything or anybody in the process. Trees produce fruit, then a perfectly designed chain of events follows: people eat, birds eat, little animals eat. That is the true meaning of sustainability. That means less pollution transporting fruit from the south (which by the time it reaches our kitchens it looses most of its enzymes), less demand on those farmers, and less pesticides are sprayed because there would be no need to force nature to produce triple than what it's actually designed to produce.

Plant an organic or non-GMO fruit tree on your front yard today, and don't use any herbicides or insecticides. You can also encourage your neighbors to do the same. Then, a couple of years down the road when your trees have matured, have a harvesting street party; play a little music, and swap fruits with your neighbors.

Raw and sprouted vegetables

The human body is an extremely intricate machine with thousands of sophisticated processes taking place from head to toe 24 hours a day. However, none of these processes— none whatsoever— would be possible if it wasn't for a bunch of little guys called *enzymes*. Enzymes are so paramountly important, without them the human body would literally cease to exist.

Enzyme pioneer Dr. Edward Howell concludes that we were born with a certain reserve of enzymes— the more you eat foods that lack in natural enzymes, the more your body turns to the existing reserves in order to sustain its biological functions. Again, the body cannot survive without enzymes. So ideally, you want as much as possible to keep the ones you have, while supplementing with naturally occurring enzymes found in raw foods (also called *living foods*). Fruits and vegetables are easiest to consume in raw form.

Then there are sprouts and microgreens, which are some of the most nutrient dense, truly life-giving foods on the planet.

Today you can find a wide variety of organic sprouts and microgreens in most grocery stores, such as onions, broccoli, red clover, peas, barley, radish, mustard, arugula, alfalfa, kamut, lentils, fenugreek, sunflower, wheat grass, beans, etc. You can also grow them yourself; it doesn't take much space and it's quite easy to do. Sprouting jars are now available on the market for around $10.00, and the cost of organic or non-GMO seeds, grains, and beans is less than what you would be spending on already grown sprouts. Aside from that, you'll start looking at food differently; there is no better feeling than to see such an unassuming, minuscule seed come to life in a few days, and turn to be such a powerhouse of enzymes.

Raw fruit and vegetables, sprouts and microgreens deliver miraculous enzymes that help the body function at its very best, all of which are destroyed during the cooking process. When you make raw food part of your daily eating habits, you'll also spend less time preparing your meals. For a healthy and very tasty salad, mix different sprouts and microgreens along with diced onion, graded carrot, olive oil, sea salt (or Himalayan) and lemon juice (or apple cider vinegar). Make a habit of eating this salad for lunch or dinner along with the protein of your choice, and you'd be doing a massive favor to your body.

Vegetables and Fruit in a nutshell:

- Non-GMO or organic are best
- Buy fruit and vegetables in season & freeze them
- Ferment vegetables
- Grow some of your own
- Plant an organic or non-GMO fruit tree
- Add raw and sprouted vegetables with meals

Fats

Full-fat

I consider the low-fat "movement" one of the most deceptive ideas of our time. Studies now show that defatted foods can damage the way your body naturally processes fats and sugar, making you actually much more prone to overeating. They can also create what scientists are now discovering an addictive behavior, which keeps you craving the wrong kind of foods. Next, because de-fatting foods strips them of their natural good taste, food additives are added to make up for the lack of taste, which can further affect one's weight and health.

Take dairy foods for example, one of the most defatted food groups. The fat in dairy is there for a very good reason, which is to balance the natural sugars existent in it. Without the fat we basically only get the sugar, which leads to spikes in the insulin levels.

Olive oil

Rich in monounsaturated fatty acids, vitamins, minerals, and antioxidants, the benefits of high-quality olive oil are countless. It helps lower the risk of heart disease, stroke, breast cancer, type 2 diabetes, and studies show it may even help in preventing gallstones. It can decrease severe pain and stiffness in people suffering of rheumatoid arthritis, and the American Diabetes Association showed in a study that a diet high in monounsaturated fat contributes to belly fat loss.

Olive oil has beauty benefits as well; it can improve skin elasticity when applied topically and has deep conditioning properties when applied 15 to 30 minutes before washing your hair.

Although olive oil has a medium smoke point, which means it can be cooked at low to medium heat, I never cook with it. Instead, I pour it over at the end when the food is off the stove. One of my favorite ways of having olive oil is on a slice of toast along with hot pepper, Himalayan salt and turmeric, which turns a boring piece of toast into a tasty source of anti-inflammatory elements.

To make sure you get all the healthy benefits of olive oil, opt for cold pressed brand stored in a dark glass bottle. The better olive oil leaves a slight peppery aftertaste at the back of the tongue.

Nuts and seeds

Consumed in moderation, almonds, peanuts, hazelnuts, pecans, cashews, sunflower, sesame, quinoa, chia, flax and pumpkin seeds, walnuts, brazil and macadamia nuts, are all great sources of healthy fats. The best way to enjoy the true benefits of nuts and seeds is by soaking them first. Nuts and seeds contain phytic acid and enzyme inhibitors, which prevent the seed from sprouting prematurely. These enzyme inhibitors can cause problems by contributing to nutrient deficiencies and irritation of the digestive system. Phytic acid binds to minerals in the digestive system, which stops nutrients from being absorbed and reduces the digestibility of nuts and seeds. By soaking them you turn a dormant, potentially problematic food into a pool of health benefiting nutrients.

Put nuts and seeds into a mason jar with water overnight. In the morning rinse, drain, and refrigerate in an airtight container. Rinse them once a day so they don't catch mold, and consume within 3 to 4 days. Use them over salads or together with a fruit, for a complete meal/snack that will not spike your insulin levels.

Avocados

The monounsaturated fats in avocados help raise the good cholesterol while lowering the bad one. Avocados are also loaded with vitamin E, which helps keep your skin young, boost immunity, and prevent damage caused by free radicals. Although consuming avocado comes with tremendous health benefits, it is still high in fat and needs to be enjoyed in moderation. It works best especially when combined with a variety of fresh greens; usually one-half of an avocado in a fresh salad is more than enough to reap the benefits of this super food.

Fats in a nutshell:

- From grass fed, hormones & antibiotic free animals, or organic
- Olive oil (cold pressed)— avoid cooking with it, best consumed cold
- Avocado, grapeseed, peanut, canola, sunflower oils — best for cooking
- Nuts and seeds— soak overnight and refrigerate
- Avocado fruit— use in salads, shakes.

Fish

Wild or organic

The first thing to keep in mind when it comes to fish is that big fish like tuna, swordfish, and shark contain the most contaminants, such as mercury. Wild sockeye salmon and Coho are next in line, while small fish like sardines and anchovies have the least amounts of toxic contaminants. Reason being, the longer the fish live, the more contaminants they accumulate in their system.

Another reason to choose organic or wild fish is because farmed fish is usually fed with corn gluten, ground-up feathers, soybean, chicken fat, genetically engineered ingredients, astaxanthin (a color added to enhance the pinkness of their flesh), antibiotics and anti-parasitic drugs to kill the sea lice. These are considered by experts unsafe for human consumption. Aside from that, fish farming puts strain on our environment by leaking toxins in our water, contaminating the marine life.

All that sounds complicated, so this is how I simplified eating fish: when it comes to bigger fish like salmon and tuna, get the organic or at least wild. Watch when they're on clearance, get a bunch and freeze them. In general, it's better to stick to small fish such as sardines, anchovies, and smelts. In many instances, they are conveniently packed in jars, which makes it very easy to be used in salads.

If you'd like to simplify further, focus on salmon and sardines, which are some of the highest in omega-3 fatty acids.

Seafood

Who doesn't like shrimp, octopus, or calamari? I do too, but the only time I truly enjoy eating them is when they are freshly caught and cooked in a modest restaurant by the sea somewhere. Other than that, I eat them very rarely, mostly at Christmas, when my Italian mother-in-law prepares her finger lickin' seafood dishes that nobody in their right mind could resist. Just make sure, especially when you eat fried seafood, that you have raw vegetables and/or salad. This way you supply your body with those amazing enzymes that help break down the food easier.

Fish in a nutshell:

- Wild or organic
- Consume bigger fish in moderation
- Smaller fish is best

Grains

Bread— Non-GMO or organic & free of additives

When someone asks me if there is a particular food I'd recommend to start with when switching to simple foods, I answer with a question: "What do you eat most of?" And the answer is almost always the same: "Bread". Bread is one of the most commonly used foods; we make sandwiches, have it as toast, French toast, we love spreading butter on it, dip it in olive oil or tomato sauce, even eat it on its own. We should not have to give it up in order to be healthy. I happen to think that the crusty, fresh out-of-the-oven bread is quite comforting.

It is said that bread increases blood sugar levels, but that's not the concern I have with bread; mamutza had bread every single day with every meal and never complained of being lethargic or tired after she ate. (Not to mention she maintained her svelte figure her whole life.) If you eat white bread alone yes, it can increase your blood sugar. However, when it's combined with healthy fiber, protein and fats, it becomes an entirely different story.

There are countless types of breads available at the grocery store, which makes finding a truly healthy version one of the most daunting experiences I personally had to go through. The problem with commercial bread is that they have 2 possibly negative aspects we have to take into consideration: the kind of flour used to make the bread, and the additives added during the production process.

When it comes to the kind of flour the bread is made with, ideally you should choose one made with non-GMO or organic flours. This will also help avoid a harmful additive called Potassium Bromate (or its derivative Bromine), which is used to bleach flour and make the dough more elastic.

However, here in Canada I'm thrilled to see some bread manufacturers are finally showing signs of understanding the importance of eating simple foods and stipulate "non-GMO" on their packages.

The second aspect I mentioned earlier is the additives used during the process of making the bread. It's always a good idea to read the ingredients even of organic bread, as commercial breads may contain: potassium bromate, azodicarbonamide, sugar, L-cysteine, high fructose corn syrup, caramel coloring, yeast nutrients, Butylated Hydroxyanisole (BHA), mono and diglycerides, ethoxylated mono and diglycerides, yeast nutrients, calcium propionate, soybean oil, soy lecithin, corn oil, soy flour, and/or corn starch. Even though it may be claimed that these additives are in *"Too small amounts to cause any harm"*, due to the fact that we eat bread for breakfast, lunch and dinner, over the years they accumulate in the body and increase the toxicity levels.

So how do I keep eating bread simple? Again, I think of my mamutza. Bread was always on her table, but it was made with unbleached wheat, baking yeast, salt, and water.

Bake some of your own bread and sweets

Making bread occasionally is not only a good choice health-wise. but it could be fun for the entire family to participate (plus your house will smell great!) There is a plethora of organic and non-GMO flours on the market today. From unbleached, whole and light spelt, oat and rye, each come with their own unique nutritional benefits. By making your own bread and sweets you save money, and your family will eat much healthier. Again, bread is one food we eat almost every single day, sometimes multiple times a day, so it becomes very important to make sure you have the right kind.

Pasta

Pasta made with white flour, spelt, brown rice, rye, buckwheat, corn, are all healthy choices provided they are made of organic or non-GMO flours, and contain no additives. Then pair it up with good fats and proteins.

Rice, barley, spelt, buckwheat, wheat

I don't consider white rice unhealthy; when paired with protein, fiber, fats and a little bit of cumin (which helps with digestion), white rice can be a nutritious side dish to any meal. Aside from rice, other grains like barley, spelt, wheat, and buckwheat are nutrient rich. They can be prepared as a side dish, adding variety and extra nutrition to your meals.

Another great way to enjoy these grains is when they're sprouted. (I mentioned before the massive health benefits that come with eating live foods.) I put whole barley, wheat or spelt kernels in water for a couple of days, change the water once a day, then put them in the fridge once sprouted. Then I use these sprouted grains in salads and sandwiches.

Oats (steel cut, flakes, etc)

I added oats on their own here because I consider their health benefits tremendous. Oatmeal is one of the best head starts you can give your body every day, provided it's made the right way. Eating the store bought, instant oatmeal filled with food additives is not the best choice. It takes roughly 10 to 15 minutes to cook your own oatmeal from scratch but if you soak your oats overnight, they will soften and cook even quicker.

Put 1/2 cup of oats and 1 cup of water in a pot, throw in any nuts and dried fruit (choose from almonds, walnuts, flax seeds, sesame seeds, chia seeds, cranberries, raisins, dates, etc), and let them soak overnight. In the morning simply turn on the stove at low-medium and cook for 5 minutes. Soaking the nuts and dried fruit makes them easier to digest and unlocks their powerful nutrients. In this form alone, oatmeal contains all elements for a perfect breakfast. However, if you have the extra minute and feel adventurous, go ahead and mix in fresh fruit, cinnamon, and a drizzle of honey.

In my opinion, this is one of the best breakfasts you can have. It will start your day with a balanced insulin.

Grains in a nutshell:

- All organic or non-GMO & free of additives
- Bread— bake some of your own bread and sweets
- Pasta— any flour, pair up with fats and protein
- Rotate various grains such as rice, barley, spelt, buckwheat, and wheat
- Sprout grains and use raw in salads and sandwiches
- Oats— soak overnight along with nuts and/or seeds, enjoy with fresh fruit for breakfast

---

Dairy

From organic, or at least grass fed and ormone & antibiotic free animals

Like meats, if your dairy doesn't come from organic or at least grass fed and hormone & antibiotic free animals, you can be ingesting toxins that your body doesn't favor. As an example, the hormone rBGH is a genetically engineered artificial hormone injected into dairy cows to increase milk production. It has been banned in 30 countries, including Canada. Health risks associated with ingestion of dairy products containing rBGH are colorectal, prostate, and breast cancers.

Full-fat, plain, and free of additives

Stick to dairy products that are in as close to their natural state as possible— full-fat, plain, and free of additives. Being considered high in saturated fats which are said to increase the bad cholesterol, dairy products have been taking serious beatings from all directions for quite some time now. If you ask me though, the only dairy I personally consider health damaging is the one that is messed around with in the lab. As long as it's enjoyed in moderation, there is absolutely no reason to be terrified of eating full-fat yogurt, or a piece of full-fat cheese. The answer to keeping fat at bay is not in messing around with what nature created, but in being smart; by eating in moderation and learning how to combine the foods, so that we keep the insulin levels steady and not store much fat.

Milk— when it comes to the subject of milk in North America there is one sensitive issue we're faced with, which is consumption of raw milk. In the U.S., raw milk is already available in many states, which I consider a huge step in the right direction. In Canada on the other hand, selling raw milk is illegal across the country, so manufacturers have to pasteurize it. The problem with pasteurization is that it destroys enzymes and beneficial bacteria, health-nurturing proteins are transformed into unnatural versions that actually promote health problems, and vitamins are greatly diminished.

Aside from pasteurization, homogenization is yet another process milk is subjected to in factories. The reason for homogenization is to break down fat into tiny particles. This gives the milk a smooth consistency, without fat particles swimming around or gathering at the top. The problem with this is that fat particles become oxidized and rancid, which is not very far from the negative health effects modified milk ingredients give. Through homogenizing, the protein in milk becomes hard to digest, thus bypassing into the blood stream. This may cause autoimmune disorders such as diabetes and multiple sclerosis.

Pasteurization and homogenization are so detrimental, that once the milk is subjected to these processes it becomes a burden on the body, even if it is organic.

Raw milk, on the other hand, contains natural enzymes, fatty acids, vitamins and minerals, making it truly a complete food. Its health benefits are vast: it reduces allergies, boosts the immune system, improves skin conditions such as psoriasis and eczema, it supports skin's hydration, prevents nutrient deficiencies, acts as a neurological support, and assists with weight loss. Raw milk contains naturally occurring sugar that the body breaks down easily, as opposed to pasteurized and homogenized milk in which harmful artificial sweeteners have to be added to make up for the lack of taste— this alone can cause a list of bothersome ailments.

The argument with raw milk is that it might contain harmful bacteria like Salmonella and E. coli. Then again, so might sprouts, mushrooms, nut butters, flavored water, oysters and other shellfish, canned chili peppers, commercial prepared teas, garlic powder, seeds, nuts, soft cheese, as well as fresh and processed meats. There have been hundreds of recalls on many products such as these— some of which made people sick— yet none of them were banned or made illegal countrywide.

One fact I can say is that I grew up drinking raw milk, and in the 24 years that I've lived in Romania I don't remember ever hearing of anybody getting sick from it. I'm hoping that one day our Canadian officials in charge of such decisions will understand that the benefits of drinking raw milk by far outweighs the "danger" of getting sick. And that sooner rather than later, people will be allowed to make their own decisions as to whether they choose to take advantage of the incredible, particularly unique benefits this white liquid gold truly has to offer.

Until we get to the historical point where raw milk is available in grocery stores indiscriminately across all North America, I would recommend purchasing organic milk that's non-homogenized, full-fat, and plain.

Kefir— the healthiest way of enjoying your dairy, aside from raw milk. For those who have never tasted it, my description of kefir is a lightly effervescent, liquidy yogurt. There is a legend saying that in the Northern region of the Caucasus, Mohammed gave kefir grains to Orthodox Christians and taught them how to make it. The kefir grains, which resemble small clumps of cauliflower, are added to fresh milk and left at room temperature. From that point, two things happen: the live grains ferment the milk turning it into kefir, and they multiply. It is this multiplication process that allows people to continually share the grains. In those times, having kefir grains was considered part of the wealth of the family, and so they were secretly passed from one generation to the next.

The method of making kefir was kept secret until the 19th century, when it was finally disclosed. News spread that kefir was successful in the treatment of tuberculosis as well as intestinal and stomach diseases. At this point Russian doctors began studying its properties, with the first studies on the benefits of kefir being published at the end of the 19th century. Up to today, the people living in the Caucasus region are known for their longevity and many accredit this to their regular consumption of kefir.

Kefir was used in the former USSR for treatment of gastrointestinal disorders, allergies, metabolic conditions, tuberculosis, atherosclerosis and cancer. Further scientific studies have been done, and kefir was proven to stimulate the immune system, inhibit tumors, fungi, and bacteria such as Helicobacter pylori. Kefir is also easily digestible, and in most cases it can be enjoyed even by those who are lactose intolerant. It contains naturally occurring probiotics, the beneficial bacteria that promotes digestive health, similar to fermented vegetables.

The benefits of consuming kefir regularly are remarkable, especially when it is made of raw (unpasteurized) milk, and it is consumed in its plain, full-fat form. However, in the absence of Kefir from raw milk, the next best thing is the pasteurized version. Just make sure it's non-homogenized, full-fat and *unflavored*. Flavored kefir (and yogurt for that matter) contains additives such as sweeteners, which are known to destroy the beneficial bacteria in it. Since the very reason to drink kefir and yogurt is mostly for their beneficial probiotics, it defeats the purpose to consume one that has none.

If you have never tasted kefir you might find it strange when you first do so, only because your taste buds are not accustomed to it. But no matter how much you dislike it, once you keep trying it your taste buds will get the message, and sooner than you think you'll have acquired the habit of liking it. My husband tasted kefir for the first time when we met, and I think it's safe to say that he absolutely hated it. But he kept trying it and today Kefir is one of his favorite drinks.

Yogurt— the next best thing after kefir, yogurt should also be consumed in its natural form: full-fat, plain, with no additives. Commercial flavored yogurts may contain artificial sweeteners, sugar or high fructose corn syrup, colors and/or preservatives, which make up a hostile environment in which their natural friendly bacteria (probiotics) cannot survive. As a result, they don't contain nearly the amount of probiotics you'd expect. In order for the friendly bacteria to survive, yogurt has to be kept in an as close to its natural form as possible— and that's full-fat and plain.

You can easily create your healthy version of the flavored yogurt by putting a layer of your favorite jam at the bottom of a cup and plain yogurt on top. This way you not only create a healthier but also more affordable version of the commercial flavored yogurt. My daughter has been making her own version of fruit yogurt since she was 4 years old. I, on the other hand, enjoy my plain yogurt drizzled with a little honey.

Cheese— according to experts, cheese is filled with nutrients that help the bones, heart, and brain, provided it is free of additives. Out of all dairy products, cheese is the one that tends to contain the most additives. For this reason, I get the ones made from raw milk (lucky it is available) and contain no additives. There is a very limited selection of simple cheeses which, in a way, makes it easy to shop once you know which ones they are.

Soy, rice, almond, coconut, and any other wanna-be milks I might've overlooked— I personally avoid them. These so-called "milks" try to emulate the taste of dairy, which is impossible. In an attempt to do so, many artificial ingredients are added. I am yet to find soy, rice, almond, or coconut milk in a form that has no dubious ingredients. However, if you're lactose intolerant, I would choose the ones that have the least additives; brown rice milk is one that I would gravitate toward.

Ice cream— one of the most beloved foods that unfortunately always contains additives, even the organic versions. If your family members love ice cream as much as mine, investing in an ice cream machine would be a very good idea not only health-wise, but from a financial standpoint as well.

If you live in an area where you have access to raw milk then what can I say, hats off to you! If you don't, use pasteurized milk but make sure that at least it's organic and non-homogenized. Remember, I don't suggest becoming a robot. Homemade, additive-free ice cream made with organic, pasteurized, non-homogenized milk is by far a much better choice than the store-bought ice cream.

You might or might not be surprised to hear that making ice cream is one of the simplest desserts to make; milk and/or cream, brown sugar, and vanilla— that is ALL you need to make your own vanilla ice cream. You can use this as a base and turn it into your favorite flavor: for strawberry ice cream add crushed strawberries; for chocolate add your favorite crushed chocolate; add a drop of mint essential oil for a refreshing mint flavor; chop up your favorite cookies and add it in.

One of my family's favorite is espresso ice cream. I make espresso coffee, sweeten and chill it, then I pour it in the ice cream machine a few minutes before the vanilla ice cream is done.

Dairy in a nutshell:

- Grass fed or organic, and from hormone & antibiotic free animals
- Milk, Kefir, Yogurt, Cheese— raw (if available), non-homogenized, full-fat, plain, no additives
- Soy, rice, almond, coconut milk, and other wanna-be milks— unless with no additives, better to be avoided
- Ice cream— make your own

Meat

Organic, or grass fed and free of hormones & antibiotics

There are quite a few reasons we should only eat meats that are organic, or at least from animals that have been grass fed and were not given hormones and antibiotics.

Hormones and antibiotics in meats— I can't even begin to express how important it is to eat meats free of hormones and antibiotics. In a recent report, Consumers Union determines *"Approximately 80 percent of the antibiotics sold in the United States are used in meat and poultry production. The vast majority is used on healthy animals to promote growth, or prevent disease in crowded or unsanitary conditions."* *"Consumers Union has concluded that the threat to public health from the overuse of antibiotics in food animals is real and growing. Humans are at risk both due to potential presence of superbugs in meat and poultry, and to the general migration of superbugs into the environment, where they can transmit their genetic immunity to antibiotics to other bacteria, including bacteria that make people sick."*

This piece of information alone should be enough to make you think twice about the kind of meats you decide to feed your kids.

Ractopamine— a drug given to animals to increase protein synthesis and make the animal more muscular. Still used in the U.S., ractopamine is banned in over 160 countries.

Chlorine— chicken is doused in chlorine to kill off germs. Chlorine is a pesticide that basically kills living organisms, which means it also can destroy cells and tissue inside our bodies. *"... the chlorine problem is similar to that of air pollution"*, Dr. Robert Carlson, researcher at University of Minnesota states. *"...chlorine is the greatest crippler and killer of modern times!"*

Phosphates— often added to meat in order to enhance color, flavor, and moisture absorption. Phosphate is an arterial toxin known to increase heart disease.

Irradiated meat— a method of preservation through exposure to low levels of radiation, prevents food borne illnesses. Not allowed in the European Union, as it changes the chemical composition of the food.

Limit intake of processed meats

The International Agency for Research on Cancer (IARC), the cancer agency of the World Health Organization, has classified processed meat as a carcinogen. Processed meats include but are not limited to bacon, hot dogs, sausages, and deli meats. Most processed meats contain nitrates, which you might or might not be surprised to learn that they are also sometimes used as fertilizers and rocket propellant. They have been controversially linked to leukemia, colon, bladder, and pancreatic cancer. Nitrates in particular may trigger migraines, while sodium nitrates may cause oxygen deprivation of the fetus in pregnant women.

You don't have to give up on your occasional bacon and eggs breakfast, but it would be wise to choose the bacon without sodium nitrites and nitrates. I know cost is an important issue when it comes to healthier meats, but think of it this way: when you spend more money on bacon that is organic, hormone & antibiotic free, sodium nitrates and nitrates free, use it as an incentive to eat a "decent" amount. By that I mean eat what your body needs, not what your habit wants.

Eat less meat

Again, organic and hormone & antibiotics free meats are more expensive, but on the other hand we generally eat far too much meat. All a person needs at one meal is the size and thickness of the palm of their hand. Anything more than that is a waste of money, even though it may not seem that way. Not to mention that you're putting an extra load on your digestive and other bodily systems. Energy that would otherwise go to the brain and other important organs, is taken away to digest the extra food.

Instead of overeating meat, fill up on vegetables; you'll feel lighter and more energetic.

Meat in a nutshell:

- Organic, or grass fed and free of hormones & antibiotics
- Limit intake of processed meats
- Eat less meat

Herbs and Spices

Herbs

Herbs add an extra dimension to foods, not only taste wise but in the form of nutritional value as well. Take parsley for example; it's loaded with Vitamin K as well as Vitamins D, B12, and A. This helps keep your immune system strong, helps your bones, heart and nervous system, it has antioxidant and anti-inflammatory properties, and with regular long-term use it even helps control your blood pressure. Herbs are truly powerhouses of nutrients, and they don't have to be consumed in high quantities in order to get their fabulous benefits.

Herbs are simple to grow; get a few small containers, add organic soil, organic seeds, and place them by a window in your kitchen. You don't have to complicate yourself with exotic herbs; parsley, rosemary, basil, mint, and thyme, are enough to not only add incredible nutritional value to your meals, but make your kitchen look and smell nice too. Chicken, turkey, or lamb thrown in the oven with only sea salt and a small rosemary branch will have an incredible aroma and taste. Parsley goes with almost any dish imaginable; simply cut it and throw it over your pastas, soups, or steak. Basil goes beautifully in tomato sauce and raw in your salads. But when it comes to how to use herbs, forget the rules. Just throw them over your food; you decide what you like and what you don't.

Spices

When it comes to spices, I don't think there are any that don't come with some sort of health benefits. However, today we are particularly faced with an epidemic of digestive system inflammation. Inflammation is already known to be the root of most if not all diseases, including cancer. David M. Marquis, Diplomat from the American Clinical Board of Nutrition says the following about inflammation: *"One could also argue that without inflammation most diseases would not even exist."*

For this reason, I decided to simplify it and focus on spices that improve the health of the digestive system. These particular spices are turmeric, caraway seeds, and garlic (depending on how it's being used, garlic is considered a vegetable or spice, but I took the liberty of categorizing it as a spice here).

Turmeric— with its powerful compound Curcumin, is known for its incredible anti-inflammatory qualities. Dr. Josh Axe, a certified doctor of natural medicine, doctor of chiropractic and clinical nutritionist says in a report *"Turmeric, the main spice in curry, is arguably the most powerful herb on the planet at fighting and potentially reversing disease." "...curcumin, is among the most effective anti-inflammatory compounds in the world."*

I use turmeric in my shakes, on toast with olive oil, as well as in my home-made macaroni and cheese.

Caraway seeds— used in Ayurvedic medicine for gastrointestinal problems among other conditions, caraway seeds have been shown to help with ailments in the digestive track such as constipation, IBS, flatulence, colic, ulcers, and high cholesterol. The antioxidants present in caraway seeds (cryptoxanthin, beta carotene, and lutein) protect against cellular damage by hunting free radicals in the body, and reduce the risk for gastrointestinal cancer.

Garlic— high in Allicin, a Sulphur compound, garlic has numerous health benefits with one of them being a natural antibiotic. When we used to get a cold, the flu, or any kind of upper respiratory infection, my mamutza used to make us swallow a clove of raw garlic clove every day. Garlic boosts the function of the immune system, it reduces blood pressure and LDL cholesterol, and it contains antioxidants that may help reduce Alzheimer's disease and dementia. The sulfur compounds in garlic have even been shown to protect against organ damage from metal toxicity. Garlic is also a pre-biotic, which helps your gut microflora flourish. When I cook, I usually add raw crushed garlic at the very end, as well as I mix it in raw vegetable dishes and salads.

Herbs and Spices in a nutshell:

- Use more herbs in your cooking
- Grow some of your own
- Add Turmeric, Garlic or Caraway seeds in your meals daily

Salt

Salt keeps your body in proper mineral balance, and just like water, it's needed by every cell in your body. However, table salt is not ideal. Aside from potentially containing particles of sand and glass which are responsible for creating small tears in the veins, it has additives like fluoride, anti-caking agents, and/or aluminium derivatives. These additives turn table salt downright toxic.

Celtic salt, Sea salt, and Himalayan salts on the other hand support your health when consumed in moderation. They contain minerals that fill the body with powerful electrolytes to keep you hydrated, and have trace elements needed for proper immune support.

Salt in a nutshell:

- Use Celtic, Himalayan, and Sea salts

Sweeteners

Raw and **brown sugar** are better choices than white granulated sugar. Pure **maple syrup** and **unpasteurized honey** are two other very good choices. They all should be organic or at least non-GMO, and consumed in moderation.

Sweeteners in a nutshell:

- Use brown sugar, pure maple syrup and unpasteurized honey

Beverages

Tea

All herbal teas are, to a certain degree, health supportive. Green tea in particular (or its powdered form

Matcha) is very high in antioxidants but not everybody enjoys its taste, including yours truly. However, because I know it has tremendous health benefits, I make it tastier by sweetening it with honey or maple syrup.

Any herbal tea has some sort of health benefits, particularly when consumed on a regular basis. For example, chamomile tea has been used for centuries as a mild, relaxing sleep aid, for stomach ailments, as well as an anti-inflammatory. Peppermint tea improves digestion, helps eliminate inflammation, relaxes the body and mind, can aid in weight loss and boosts the immune system. St. John's Wort tea acts as a mild antidepressant and has antibacterial, anti-viral, anti-inflammatory and antioxidant properties. And the list goes on.

Think of what bothers you: are you experiencing headaches, acid reflux, constipation, or irritability? Do your research and find what herbal tea might help with your particular health issue, and make a habit of drinking it daily. If you can't think of any (God bless!), then choose a herbal tea that you might want to consume as a preventative measure, or simply because it's comforting.

Regardless of what herbal tea you decide to drink regularly, in the long run it will have beneficial effects on your body.

Coffee

Based on scientific research, coffee is rich in beneficial antioxidants; it increases brain alertness, boosts the metabolism, improves physical performance, may lower the risk of type II diabetes, dementia, Alzheimer's and Parkinson's diseases, and may even lower risk of some types of cancers. Drinking coffee daily is not the problem.

The problem is when the coffee you drink is not organic, and it's filled with refined sugar and creamer.

Today you can find organic or fair-trade coffee at your local wholesale store, and the good news is it will not cost you as much as you usually pay at the coffee shop daily. I understand the feeling of getting your coffee from your favorite coffee shop, and I do too once in a while. But try to break that daily habit and turn it into a sporadic event instead. You will not only enjoy better health but save money in the process as well.

Juice & Soda

Most commercial juices and sodas, including the "healthy" versions, are pasteurized. That means they lack the necessary enzymes that aid in the digestion process and so the body has to work harder to break them down. They are also filled with added ingredients like sugar, fructose, food coloring, artificial sweeteners, and/or the infamous *natural flavor*. These are all harmful to the body, especially when consumed on a regular basis. I believe any kind of pasteurized juice—organic or not— doesn't support the wellbeing of any *body*.

Although I don't consider soda much different than most commercial juices in the sense that neither improves the wellbeing of the human body, it is still a step down from juice. Sodas tend to contain a higher amount of harmful food additives, such as Bromine, a substance used in some flours. These additives are banned in Europe and Japan.

Unsweetened and unpasteurized juices are best choices, as they contain real vitamins, minerals and enzymes.

Alcohol

We all know having a glass of red wine can be beneficial for the heart and arteries, but what about white wine? I was actually surprised to find out that white wine has equal benefits as red wine. While red wine gets its fame due to its Resveratrol content, white wine is beneficial due to different components called Tyrosol and Hydroxytyrosol. These components are equally important in improving heart function and preventing artery blockage. Dipak K. Das, a professor at the University of Connecticut School of Medicine led a study on white wine and got to the conclusion that white wines contain an antioxidant similar to the one found in olive oil.

However, most commercial wines come with added sulfites, a preservative intended to prevent oxidization and maintains freshness. Sulfites might be beneficial for the wine but not so much for people. Organic wines are available, although they're quite costly. I'd suggest enjoy your wine in moderation or better yet, make your own. If you're a true wine lover who has to have that glass at dinner, investing in the right tools and making your wine once a year could be a truly gratifying experience.

Beverages in a nutshell:

- Tea— pick a herbal tea(s) that you enjoy
- Coffee— make it at home from organic or fair trade coffee beans
- Avoid pasteurized Juices & Soda— make your own
- Red and white wine— enjoy occasionally

A few last guidelines

The idea is not to fully jump into an organic, raw, home cooked diet. Remember that everything you eat on a regular basis you eat because you created a habit. It would be challenging to suddenly switch to eating 100% simple foods and be successful long-term. Start with what you consume most of on a daily basis— if it's coffee you drink every day, then start with that. Purchase your coffee organic or fair trade from one of your local wholesale vendors, and create a habit of making it at home. Take the next food most consumed by your family and replace it with the simpler, organic or non-GMO, additive-free version. And so on.

As much as possible, purchase foods that are in their original, nature-intended form— basically foods that don't come with ingredient lists attached. If you must have something in a package, check the ingredients. If it contains anything that you do not understand, I suggest avoiding it. Don't rush to assume that "yeast extract" must be yeast, because it's not— if it was yeast, it would simply say "yeast".

Eat fresh fruit before your meals— fresh fruit provide the digestive system enzymes needed to better digest whatever you're eating next. Also, eating fruit after a meal could cause fermentation and bloating— unless it's berries or pineapple, which contain enzymes that help with digestion.

If losing some of the fat deposits is the goal, you might also want to take this into consideration: temporary hunger is your friend because it helps lose fat, and it detoxifies at cellular level.

> **It helps lose fat**— if you're generally healthy with no medical conditions, let yourself be hungry once in a while. When you eat, the food is converted into glycogen and gets stored in the liver to be used for energy. Every time you eat, the liver stores glycogen to use as a main source of energy. Once that glycogen is consumed and the body doesn't receive any food, the liver will turn to existing fat deposit and start breaking them down to use for energy. But if at the first sign of hunger you grab a snack, your glycogen levels will get replenished and the liver will not have the opportunity to use your existing fats as energy.

> **It detoxifies at cellular level**— *"...create a little hunger. When we don't eat for a certain amount of time the body's recycling system will kick in, our newzymes will be activated, and the defective protein in our cells will be shredded and turned into healthy protein*", says Dr. Hiromi Shinya, the modern colonoscopic technique pioneer. By detoxifying at cellular level, your body's immune system becomes stronger and able to eliminate existing pathogens more efficiently.

I personally do a mini-fast 1-2 times per week: I stop eating at 6pm, then for the next 17 hours I only have lots of lemon water.

Chapter 5

FITNESS

WE ARE MADE TO MOVE

Weight loss is one of the hottest topics of our time. Many of us would do almost anything to lose those unwanted pounds, and FAST— the faster, the better. Of course we know that's not possible. Sure we've heard over and over that once we've completed an extreme weight loss program, the weight will come back with interest. Still, we try. We work out excessively, eat below the minimal caloric requirement, and look for the lowest fat foods we can find— all this at the very least. Some are willing to take it even further and risk their lives by taking various drugs that come with the promise of melting fat but may also cause horrifying effects such as elevated heart rate, stroke, even heart attacks.

Giuseppe and I used to own a fitness facility in a small town north-west of Toronto. We had our long-term members, but there was also an influx of new faces in the beginning of each year. Year after year we watched this bunch of eager people come first week of January, then disappear by the time March break came along. Our main goal as a fitness centre was to inspire people in our community to be active; we did everything we could to guide and teach them into maintaining and improving their levels of fitness. But seeing these people willingly enroll for a full year membership and then quit 3 months later, made us question whether we were— basically— doing our job right. Therefore, we created new programs and added extra aerobic classes, offered free fitness assessments and training sessions, added gratuitous extensions to their yearly memberships. We even went as far as putting a second mortgage on our home to build an women-only section. But no matter how much we tried, this behavior continued to happen over and over again, year after year. It eventually became clear that no perks were going to make a difference for that particular bunch of people.

Then we finally realized it was something else entirely keeping them from accomplishing their goals: a wrong mindset. They were coming in motivated by their choice— their New Year's resolutions mostly— but lacking an awareness of the being steadfast stage, which is the stage where the new positive habits are given a chance to develop and become automatic.

Having unrealistic expectations also played an important part in their quitting. Many expected to lose 20 lbs by March break, when in reality it takes longer than that to undo the overeating from Halloween, Thanksgiving, Christmas and New Year's alone!

Unfortunately, most of them seemed to be under the impression that choosing to go on extreme training routines and/or diets will bring about the results they wanted. The most common justification I heard was, *"I'll only do this temporarily until I lose these 20 pounds, and after I'll maintain by doing the right thing."* I know you want long-lasting results. I know you want to be vibrant and healthy. All that can definitely be attained however, not by working out to the extreme, by taking weight loss pills or starving yourself, then thinking that you'll do the right thing *after*.

How do you figure you're going to do "the right thing" after, when you're not educating yourself on how to do it the right way in the first place? Do you think that once you lose those extra 10, 30, or 50 pounds, you're going to miraculously know how to follow a healthy lifestyle and maintain an optimal weight? In order to keep up what you had just achieved you're still going to have to learn and educate yourself about doing it the right way. In the end you'll realize that not only did you have to adjust to a painful temporary weight loss experience but once you're done with that, you'll have to adjust to yet another program: the right one.

Going back to the bunch who usually quit by March, the following January most of them would come back with even more weight to lose. Although some they did lose some weight in the beginning, once they got off the radical programs they gained it all back, plus more in some cases.

Not realizing that fitness is a lifelong commitment is the point where failing begins. Everything you do after that, even if you work out 6 times a week, has no substance because eventually you're bound to get tired of it and give up. On the other hand, even if you do achieve your desired results, now there is a chance that you might slow down or stop working out altogether because you achieved what you wanted. (I'm aware that there are cases in which once they start a fitness routine some people might realize being active has a much deeper impact, and they continue working out even after they achieved the outcome they wanted. Unfortunately, that doesn't happen too often and obviously this chapter does not apply to those particular cases.)

Being in a hurry to achieve a certain body image can make you turn to harmful weight loss methods, which will mostly give volatile results. Extreme weight loss methods can create significant limitations and set you back from implementing a long-term healthy lifestyle. Even if you do succeed and reach your (weight) goal that way, you won't be able to sustain that kind of intensity long term. And once you attain your goal, most likely you're going to stop. Reason being, an extreme program that doesn't naturally mesh with the particularities of your lifestyle brings in extra stress. In particular, working out at high intensity without gradually building up to it can create a high amount of free radicals in your body, something called *oxidative stress*. While a little bit of oxidative stress helps the cells in your body become stronger, excessive or choric oxidative stress may actually cause cellular damage which can further cause heart disease, atherosclerosis, cancer, dementia, premature aging, even early death.

There is a lot of pressure on teenagers— girls especially— who are easily brainwashed with our modern age definition of perfection. It's old news these days that body image is very much taken into consideration— it's the first thing we see and obviously, the first thing we judge. Many of them walk around feeling inadequate, ready to do almost anything to fit in that volatile mold. Unfortunately, that doesn't only apply to young girls but adults as well— I saw it all day every day in many of the people coming through our fitness center. Working in that particular environment, I had a unique privilege of learning about people's desires, vulnerabilities, even fears, related to body image. It seemed like each person had different reasons to spend money on a gym membership, but the underlining desire of most of them was to look good. There is absolutely nothing wrong with wanting to look good— but only if the subject of your goal is a better version of *you*, and not some Photoshop offspring you saw in a magazine.

In fitness, as with anything else, the kind of mindset you adopt makes the difference in whether the effects will be long-lasting or even achieved. A goal that in my opinion has the capacity to keep anyone truly motivated is to enjoy long-lasting wellness. Now this is a completely different approach. The right mindset views fitness as means to feel better— have a strong heart, a toned muscular system and good flexibility, so that they're not limited by unnecessary, sometimes debilitating pains. The beauty is that a nice-looking body is always a byproduct of a healthy lifestyle.

Once you make being healthy your main goal, you will automatically choose right— you will not engage in energy depleting workouts, become obsessed with working out and create an imbalance in your life. The right mindset will not have unrealistic expectations such as "I will lose 50 pounds in 3 months". The right mindset understands that patience is an extremely important piece of the puzzle; patience truly is the best virtue to have when setting a fitness goal, or any goal for that matter.

So see, in the long run it really doesn't matter how long it takes to reach your goal— maintaining what you've accomplished will be easy now because you did it *the right way*.

The first step before deciding anything is to mentally get yourself to the point where it makes sense to choose right. Don't put yourself through double the trouble, do it right the first time. Try to think from a different perspective: how long did it take you to put on those 30 pounds? It was the result of a slow and consistent way of eating, way of moving (or not moving). You did it by creating a strong system of habits that have been working wonderfully on your behalf. You achieved it *little by little*.

Now you want to lose 30 pounds in one month. Do you think you could *gain* 30 pounds in one month? Of course not. The body is smart; it has its own defense mechanisms that won't allow you to do that. The extra weight is there to stay because you achieved it gradually. And that's exactly the way to make it come off and stay off: gradually. Think in reverse and you got the answer to losing weight for good. Just like you "patiently" gained that extra weight, now think in reverse and patiently lose that extra weight. The idea here is not to deplete your body by subjecting yourself to extreme training routines, eliminating all fats, breads and pasta from your diet. The answer to a healthy, long-lasting weight loss is to educate yourself on doing it the right way and being patient in the process. You do that, you adopt the right frame of mind, and now you're set on the right path to accomplishing your goal.

So how should you start? If you've never worked out before, if you're a proverbial couch potato, the worst thing to do in my opinion is to join a gym and hire a personal trainer. I hate to say this but it's the truth. Unless you have no cap on your finances and are able to hire the trainer indefinitely, that expensive training will not help much unless it also teaches you the very basics. By "basics" I don't mean "Do cardio 3-5 times per week and strength training 2-3 times per week". What I'm talking about here is the basics that form the foundation of a healthy lifestyle in general— learning how to successfully eliminate bad habits and create long-lasting positive ones. Habits can't be created or broken overnight, so my suggestion is to start from the basics and build on it. It's the simple habitual things that you engage in regularly that create and sustain the right "picture" in the long run.

To give you an example here, my husband is a big advocate of the 15-minute workout. His argument is that if a 160-pound person jogs for 15 minutes 4 times per week, they'd be working out a total of 52 hours over the course of 1 year. Considering they'd be burning roughly 145 calories per workout, that translates into more than 30,000 calories being burnt in 1 year, or the equivalent of roughly 8.6 pounds of fat. In a nutshell, if you didn't overeat and worked out only 15 minutes 4 times per week, by the end of the year you would have lost anywhere between 8 to 9 pounds.

As you can see, it all adds up.

Here is the order of steps I recommend for someone who's never worked out before and is looking to improve their overall flexibility, muscle tone, and cardiovascular system. The 5th step becomes important if you want to take it to the next level, so it's totally up to you whether you decide to do it.

Take one step at a time, making sure you turn each one into a habit. Should you feel more adventurous, start with the first couple of steps at the same time, but no more than that.

As you go through each step, try not to look at it as something "outside of you" that you have to constantly adjust your life to. It has to come to the point where each step is naturally part of you and your schedule, just like eating and sleeping. When you get to the point where you see working out as part of who you are and what you normally do, you've created the habit. Then you can move on to the next step.

Here are the 5 steps:
- Stretch
- Keep It Moving
- Take It Outside
- Up A Notch— Follow a Workout Routine
- Hiring a Personal Trainer

Stretch

If you completely and utterly don't want to work out, you should at least consider stretching. Regardless of whether your job involves sitting for prolonged periods of time or you have a physically demanding job, stretching is equally (and vitally) important.

Stretching is the most natural thing to do. Look at babies, look at cats and dogs; the first thing they do when they wake up is stretch. Stretching improves the overall condition of your body. It increases muscle control and range of motion, it relaxes your muscles and releases endorphins (the hormones that promote a general good feeling). This will further improve your sleep, which makes stretching one of the best habits to have before going to bed at night.

Stretching, which in many instances incorporates yoga moves, can sometimes have miraculous effects on the body. Something I consider one of the most valuable outcomes of stretching is that it improves the function of the lymphatic system. The lymphatic system (the "plumbing" system that carries away waste products from every cell in the body) doesn't come equipped with a pump like the heart. That means it relies on you to keep it in motion. Aside from regular exercise, eating simple foods, managing stress, deep breathing and drinking enough fluids, one great way of helping the lymphatic system function properly is by stretching.

Many of the annoying pains creeping up once we reach our forties are not because of serious medical conditions or old age, but in many cases are the result of misusing our bodies by sitting for prolonged periods, overuse due to repetitive motions, and poor posture. To give you an example, a few years ago my right hip started hurting out of the blue. This hip would hurt me all the time: when sitting, when standing, even when I was sleeping at night. For a few seconds I was inclined to give into the common belief, "Once you reach 40...", but I quickly changed my mind. I started by analyzing my posture during the day and realized that every time I would stand, I had a bad habit of leaning on my right leg. So from that point on I made sure that every time I stood up, I balanced my body on both legs equally and held my back straight. It wasn't as easy as I thought to beat my habit of standing crooked; but I kept at it like a robot and soon enough it became second nature. To my total surprise, the hip pain went away within a couple of weeks.

Another culprit of chronic pains and aches is sitting for prolonged periods of time. Breaking down your long sitting sessions— by simply standing up every 20 minutes to walk and stretch lightly for even a few seconds— will make a significant difference in the way you feel overall.

The same applies if you have a physically demanding job involving the same repetitive movement; this can cause tensions, strain, and possibly injuries down the road. Aside from strength exercises (which I will be talking about later), many of the pains and strains due to overuse could be easily avoided if you stretch regularly. When you stretch on a consistent basis, the body releases its tensions and gently realigns itself; as a result, the aches and pains subside.

I would say stretching is the least pretentious of all forms of exercise, in the sense that it requires very little space and no equipment. You don't even have to set a time aside for it if you don't wish to; you could be watching your favorite TV show and stretch at the same time. Once you memorized your stretches, you can follow a routine without putting much attention on it.

Another upside of stretching is that in order to continuously get results you don't have to change your routine regularly, as you would with a fitness program. You could be doing the same stretches over and over for the rest of your life, and you'd still be getting excellent results— provided you do it correctly. I have put together complimentary fitness videos for the purpose of this book. For information on how to get your access code for the fitness videos, please see information on page 283. The video titled *"Habits Rule You – Stretch"* is a stretching routine I personally do every night before going to sleep. You can do this routine as an active meditation to calm your mind before going to sleep, or when you watch TV at night. Although taking some quiet time before going to bed would be ideal, either way you chose to do your stretches will give you the same awesome physical benefits.

All major muscle groups should be stretched: your abdominals, back, chest, calves, the muscles surrounding your neck, and forearms (especially if your hand is stuck to your computer mouse for extended periods of time). However, due to our inclination as Homo sapiens to be using our legs to get from one point to another (to which

we added the modern-day tendency of sitting for hours), there are 3 specific muscle groups that have a higher predisposition of getting tight and causing imbalances in the body. These muscles are:
- Hip flexors
- Hamstrings
- Glutes

Hip flexors

The hip flexor muscle group includes the muscles starting from your lower abdominals, going down to the front of your hips and pelvis, all the way down to your knees. The simple act of walking employs the hip flexors. Due to our anatomy, these are some of the most commonly used muscles in the body, so they end up being "naturally" tight. Then we take it to a higher level of tightness when working out— especially on treadmills, bikes, elliptical and rowing machines— or when we do any exercises that involve bending our legs and bringing them toward the abdomen (such as in squatting). But it doesn't stop there. It gets worse when we sit for prolonged periods of time. Sitting puts the hip flexors in a "shortened" position, which tightens them further. Depending on how long you're sitting at one time, blood circulation and nerve activity in the area is also negatively affected.

Tight hip flexors— whether from simply walking, working out, or sitting for long periods of time— will pull onto your pelvis and cause strain on your lower back and hips. A large percentage of low back pain people experience is because of tight hip flexors; something that could be taken care of by simply stretching daily for 20 seconds each side.

If you're an avid jogger, love your rowing machine (like I do), or work your lower body intensely, by all means don't stop doing it just because these activities can tighten your hip flexors. Just make sure you pay deliberate attention to these muscles by stretching them thoroughly right after your workout when your muscles are still warm.

Hamstrings

The effects of tight hamstrings are similar to those of tight hip flexors in the sense that when they're not being stretched, they pull the pelvis out of its natural alignment. This can affect your low back, hips, even the knees. Hamstrings are naturally tight and can get tighter as a result of working out and not stretching afterwards. Sitting with your legs bent for longer periods of time keeps your hamstrings in a "shortened" position, which can further decrease their flexibility.

Tight hamstrings can be loosened by gentle and regular stretching. Just pay attention whether your hamstrings hurt even though you stretch regularly. In that case, there might be a different reason for having pain going down the back of your legs (with a compressed sciatic nerve by your glutes muscles being one of the top to make the list). If you had an injury and/or suffer from chronic pain, it's always a good idea to first be assessed by a health care practitioner, who can evaluate whether personalized treatment is required.

Glutes

Your glutes, just like your hip flexors, are attached to the pelvis but are situated opposite to them. This means that together they help hold the pelvis in position (other muscles around your core help as well). When glutes and hip flexors are either weak or tight, it causes an imbalance in the body that may lead to pelvis tilt and thus low back strain. The attention you give to your hip flexors— in the form of strengthening and stretching— should equally be given to your glutes, so that a balance is achieved between the 2 muscle groups. As I mentioned before, sitting for longer periods tightens your hip flexors. If you look at the muscles opposite to them— your glutes— they would be in a stretched position. Over-stretching due to prolonged sitting can make them weak. This can further weaken your core, your abdominal and spinal muscles, and can cause trouble in the lower back. Someone who sits down for a long period of time should definitely strengthen and stretch both glutes and hip flexors, but emphasis should be put on *stretching* the hip flexors and *strengthening* the glutes.

Here are a few important points to keep in mind when stretching:
- Hold the stretches for 20 to 30 seconds. You'll get little benefits with less than 20 seconds, while stretching longer than 30 seconds may lead to injuries.
- Move very slowly when you go into a stretch, as well as when you come out of a stretch. Going into a stretch fast can cause pain and even injuries to muscle fibers. Coming out of a stretch quickly can cause cramping and pain. If the stretch involves keeping your head upside down (such as bending down to touch your toes), it can cause head rush and sometimes even faint, so be cautious when doing this stretch in particular.

- Relax the muscle that you are stretching. As you hold the stretch and focus on relaxing it, you'll notice the muscle becoming looser. This is a sign that you're doing the stretch correctly.
- Relax the opposite muscle of the muscle you are stretching. When stretching, there is a natural tendency to tense the opposite muscle, but you should focus on relaxing it. For example, when stretching your hamstrings try to relax your quad muscles (the front of your thigh). The stretch will not only feel better, but you will get better results as well.
- Keep it within the comfortable range. Do not go deeper into the stretch should you feel discomfort or pain. Although you should feel a bit of a pull, the general feeling should be of stress release and relaxation.
- Breathe deep: in through your nose filling your lungs with air, then exhale very slowly through your mouth until you feel your lungs empty. Breathing this way continuously for 5 to 10 minutes releases tension and also alleviates feelings of anxiety.

Please do not take stretching lightly— the difference between sitting on the couch when watching TV and doing gentle stretches when watching TV is considerable, to say the least.

One more thing you might want to keep in mind is that although stretching is incredibly beneficial on its own, it would be great to combine it with a regular strength training routine.

Keep It Moving

Innately, everything in our bodies is in constant motion: cells, blood, lymphatic system, heart, liver, brain, fluids in the spine, muscles... everything MOVES. This intricate system held together in perfect harmony by the largest organ— the skin— is moving within us. Therefore, SO SHOULD WE.

I don't know about other parts of the world, but here in North America the houses grow bigger and bigger every day, while we see less and less people outside. We don't move as much as we used to. We get in and out of our cars. Some of us think we are justified to take it easy the rest of the day just because we worked out at the gym. I have to admit that's what I thought too for a while. Then I learned that you could be working out at the gym regularly but if you sit down at work the rest of the day without getting up frequently, you quite literally poison your body.

According to Dr. David B. Angus, 5 or more hours of sedentary sitting is the equivalent of smoking a pack and a quarter of cigarettes. Additionally, Dr. David Coven, a cardiologist at St. Luke's Roosevelt Hospital Center says, *"Smoking certainly is a major cardiovascular risk factor, and sitting can be equivalent in many cases."*

When it comes to fitness, first thing to keep in mind is that the body wants to do what it wants to do, which is MOVE. There are many opportunities during the course of the day to do so; by being mindful of how you move and use your muscles, you can turn any boring house chore into a form of exercise. Everything that you do, do it with fitness in mind. Be glad to go up and down the stairs in your house when you need to, be glad to have to clean your house— even do it more often. Vacuum and mop your floors, clean your windows, scrub your pots and oven. Unless you have an existing injury— in which case consult your doctor first— don't shy away from lifting heavier things. Just make sure you don't bend over from the waist; use your legs by squatting, and keep your back straight. Instead of asking your child to get you a glass of water on movie night, get up and get it yourself— move, move, move.

This might sound simple but the results are far from simple. Sweating from vacuuming for 30 minutes or sweating from walking fast for 30 minutes doesn't really make a difference when it comes to the effects on the body. As a matter of fact, aside from your legs you also use more of your arms and upper body muscles when vacuuming. I'm not implying to replace walking with vacuuming; walking has its unique benefits and doing both would be ideal. But if you have to do something you're dreading on a regular basis— such as cleaning your house— you might as well change your frame of mind and make it work for you.

If your level of physical activity is minimal, I would say that moving more within your environment is the most important first step to take. Give your body what it wants. When you do that consistently, after a while change will start happening on different levels simultaneously. Since you'll be sending more oxygen-rich blood to your brain and muscles, you'll start feeling better overall and to a certain extent, you'll even improve your endurance and strength. It won't be as difficult to bend and twist, sprint up the stairs, carry that laundry basket, or mop the floors. Not only will you be in better physical shape, but you will also end up with a cleaner house— that on its own will bring more clarity and positive order in your life.

Take It Outside

A few years ago, my car was stolen and was in between cars for a period of time. As this was the summer break, I took it as an opportunity to challenge my endurance. I walked my daughter to summer camp daily, took her swimming and to the movies, even brought light groceries on our way home. Even though I was following a regular workout routine at home, when I added this new activity I started feeling so good, I began to genuinely look forward to walking. I felt I was promoted to a whole new level of endurance, a whole new level of wellness.

My mamutza had such endurance, as a teenager I could never keep up with her. She was able to walk fast for hours, while holding a sack of weeds over her back with one hand and her scythe with the other hand. She didn't have defined abs as would someone who follows a training routine but, as she was consistently in motion, she never had a weight issue or complained of major pains in her body.

This is the outcome we want— to be active in general. Then working out at the gym will take it to the next level, it will give you that extra edge.

The body doesn't care for complicated, latest technology workout machines. The body wants— simply— to move. Our ancestors never took the elevator, or the car. I'm aware that times have changed drastically, that it's unrealistic to walk everywhere. But that should make us even more vigilant about what is really happening to our health by always relying on our gas-powered wheels.

Take the old-fashioned walk every day and make it faster as you build endurance. Go hiking or take a bike ride; play sports with your kids. Take the stairs instead of the elevator, park far from the mall entrance— you're almost always guaranteed you'll find a spot at the furthest corner of the parking lot.

If you live not too far from the grocery store, get one of those wheeled carts and do adventure to walk to the grocery store on the weekends. I know everyone's very busy but think of it as part of your work out and you'll find it easier to make time for it. You'll be surprised to discover how quickly the body reacts positively to a simple change like that. Do that once a week, and by the end of the year you'll have 52 extremely simple, yet life-promoting cardio workouts under your belt, which also helped you lose some unwanted fat deposits. And let's not forget also about our resilient planet as, which for 52 days a year will have to deal with a little less pollution, just because one person— YOU— decided to walk to the grocery store once a week.

Up A Notch— Follow a Workout Routine

If you decide to work out that's great, but let me remind you to not get fooled into thinking that that's enough; it would be ideal had you first created a habit of stretching and being active in general. Some of us tend to think that it's ok if we go to the gym for an hour every day. And that's fine but it's not all the body wants— remember that sitting for 5 hours straight is equivalent to smoking more than a pack of cigarettes a day. Keeping your body moving has to become habit, one which will also be very helpful if you decide to start a workout program.

Let's assume that you're doing your stretches regularly, and you're also moving more within your environment. Now you can take it up a notch. Planning ahead for one year is a great idea, as it can help stay focused. Also, one year is a realistic time frame to achieve almost any fitness goal.

Before starting their long-term training, athletes always plan their year ahead. This is called *periodization*. Periodization is a methodical planning of physical training stretched over a specific period of time, with the main idea to reach the best possible results. Usually a year is divided into 4 periods of time, and a specific routine is followed in each period. The phases of a periodization program differ based on the athlete's particular sport. However, the 2 main important phases which are always taken into consideration are the *adaptation* and *active rest* periods.

A periodization program will always start with an adaptation phase during which the focus is on general strength and getting the muscles and tendons ready for the next phases. This prepares their bodies for the more intense phases that usually follow adaptation, such as *muscle growth* and *strength*. Active rests are also added within the program. During these active rests, various leisure activities are done; activities that are demanding enough to keep up the new conditioning level of the body, but light enough to give the body a chance to recover.

You might be wondering why I brought this into discussion— most of us don't train to become athletes! The thing is, whether you're an athlete, someone who's been working out at the gym regularly, or someone who's never lifted a weight before, our bodies need the same kind of attention. Maybe not the same intensity and details in a training program, but certain aspects should be taken into consideration regardless of one's fitness level and goal. As non-athletes we, too, could greatly benefit from planning ahead and approaching our fitness program as a one-year adventure. Therefore, we're going to divide the year into 4 phases of 12 weeks each.

Let's talk about the 3 important concepts that athletes take into consideration, concepts which we will integrate into the training routine of regular people like you and I, so that we also get excellent results ☺. These concepts are:

- Adapt
- Change
- Active Rest

Adapt— I'd like to underline the importance of first getting your body ready, as opposed to jumping directly into a high intensity training routine. Sometimes you might feel like you could do more but the reality is that your muscles, and especially your tendons, are not ready. It's important to give your body a chance to gradually get used to the new activity, particularly if you've never worked out before. This is the main reason why I never recommend hiring a personal trainer at this point. Every personal trainer's goal is to give you results and they may push it harder to get you the goals you want, regardless of whether you've never lifted a weight before in your life. I've seen it firsthand when a personal trainer (who was also a professional body builder) pushed her new female client to do such heavy weighted squats, that her client had to delay the rest of the sessions because she could not walk or sit down properly for 2 weeks. What I found even more distressing was that the trainer kept bragging about how good of a job she did, "See, my client could not even walk after I worked her out", AND her client was *buying* it— both metaphorically and literally!

A high increase in the production of lactic acid in the body, which is a byproduct of working out especially at high intensity, can lead to increased oxidative stress. Aside from the inconvenience of being in pain, increased oxidative stress could snowball into cell damage and early aging. Giving your body a chance to adapt to working out is a smart way to introduce exercising into your lifestyle and enjoy its benefits long-term.

Change— change your routine regularly. Within 2 to 3 months of regular training the body will adapt to whatever routine you're on. That means it will eventually reach a plateau point and respond less and less to your training. In other words, you won't get significant results from that point on. You should change your routine regularly, with a general rule of thumb being every 8 to 12 weeks. A new routine will surprise the body and force it to readapt, resulting in an increase in strength and endurance, as well as an improved body image.

Active Rest— once you start working out, giving your body a chance to rest becomes just as important as exercising. Small tears take place in the muscle fibers particularly during strength training, and unless you give the body the adequate time to fix them, you won't get the full benefits from your workouts. This could also cause injuries down the road. While at rest, your body goes on repairing these micro tears, and because it usually "forgets" how they were initially, it rebuilds them stronger than before. This is what ultimately causes increased strength, muscle tone, and mass.

I don't recommend working out 7 days a week. Depending on the intensity of your workouts, you need time to recover. Reserve 1 or 2 days in which you could be doing your stretches and go for walks, but refrain from actually working out. Although working out consistently 5 days a week would be ideal, for someone who's never followed a regular routine, even 3 workouts per week would be enough to make a significant difference.

Aside from the weekly 1 to 2 days of rest, it's also important to schedule 4 weeks of active rest within your year-long program. This increases the body's recovery, adds variety, and gives a sense of mental relief. During this time, regular training is replaced with activities you don't normally do: could be anything from hiking, biking, Yoga, Pilates, ballet class, to playing sports such as tennis, hockey, volleyball, soccer, and swimming— anything that is completely different than the 4 routines you have chosen. Think of this active rest period as your body's opportunity to fully craft the results for you.

Working Out at Home

There are 2 ways you can start on a training program and be equally successful: working out at home or joining a gym. Whichever way you decided to start, first plan your entire year ahead. Think of it this way: you need to schedule in 4 different workout programs of 12 weeks each, plus 2 active rests of 2 weeks each. This adds up to 52 weeks, or 1 year.

Ideally, you should first schedule in your 2 active rests. Think of when you might want to do more leisure activities as opposed to a set fitness routine. You might want this period to coincide with the Christmas holidays, your family vacation, or summer break. For example, you can plan one active rest of 2 weeks during your vacation, and the second active rest of 2 weeks during a holiday. Many people I know feel guilty after taking a vacation because they missed their workouts. Knowing that during your vacation you're actually supposed to get off your training routine and do leisure activities instead, will make the whole not-working-out experience lighter. You'll feel like you've actually accomplished more during your vacation, as opposed to being stressed out that you have to make up for the lost training when you get back. Just make sure you integrate leisure activities and sports into your daily program and actually do it. Think about how much fun you can have playing beach volleyball, walking or jogging on the beach, surfing, swimming, or hiking.

Now that you scheduled in your 2 active rests, it's time to schedule in your training routines. The following is a 1-year plan with access to fitness videos customized for each period. *(Remember to read the information on page 283 on how to get your access code for my fitness videos).*

Period 1 (12 weeks)

Keeping in mind the importance of giving your muscles and tendons a chance to adapt, start Period 1 with a less intense program that focuses on the entire body. This way your muscles and tendons have a chance to gradually tone up and get accustomed to working out.

The fitness program I created for Period 1 is titled *Habits Rule You – Period 1 – Full Body*. This program works entirely with your own body weight, without the use of any equipment.

Period 2 (12 weeks)

For the second 12-week period I created a workout that puts more emphasis on the lower body. Although this program focuses on legs and buttocks, it also works out the rest of the body. The video I created for this period is titled *Habits Rule You – Period 2 – Lower Body/Full Body*.

Period 3 (12 weeks)

For this period, I created a routine that will help increase tone and strength in the upper body, and it's titled *Habits Rule You – Period 3 – Upper Body/Full Body*. The focus here is to maintain what we have achieved so far, plus I added minimal equipment such as free weights, rubber bands, and the ball.

With this type of workout particular attention should be put on stretching your muscles. I never stretch before exercising, nor do I ever recommend it. You want to start your workout session by warming up first, then stretch during or after you work out when the muscles are warm and resilient. This will help release some of the lactic acid and toxins that usually build up within the muscles, and it will reduce post-exercise muscle soreness.

Active rest 1 (2 weeks)

During your active rest play sports outside with your kids, go hiking, bike riding, dancing— any activity that you normally wouldn't do. Just keep it moving and continue using those newly improved muscles.

Period 4 (12 weeks)

For this period, I created 2 workouts: one that focuses on the upper body titled *Habits Rule You – Period 4 – Upper Body,* and a second one which focuses on the lower body titled *Habits Rule You – Period 4 – Lower Body.* In order to properly recover, you should give your muscles a 48-hour break in between workouts. A proper weekly routine would be to alternate the 2 videos. For example, if you decide to work out 4 times a week, do the first video on Mondays and Wednesdays and the second video on Tuesdays and Thursdays.

Active rest 2 (2 weeks)

Follow the guidelines from your first active rest period.

You'll notice that all my workouts contain medium to intense core exercises. The core is your body's powerhouse not only because when it's toned it makes you feel strong and less prone to injuries, but it houses your inner organs and central nervous system. I like giving special attention to the core muscles and build both *stability* and *strength*. By building stability, the function and tone of the many little internal muscles is improved, while strength focuses more on the abdominals, obliques and low back muscles found at the superficial level.

Complete your *Keep It Moving* lifestyle by continuing to stretch at night to help your body recover from working out and keep your flexibility in check, as well as doing cardiovascular activities such as walking or jogging.

WORKING OUT AT HOME
One-Year Fitness Chart

PERIOD 1
Week 1 – Week 12
FULL BODY

- Frequency: 3-5 times/ week
- *Habits Rule You – Period 1 – Full Body* VIDEO

PERIOD 2
Week 13 – Week 24
LOWER BODY / FULL BODY

- Frequency: 3-5 times/ week
- *Habits Rule You – Period 2 – Lower Body/Full Body* VIDEO

PERIOD 3
Week 25 – Week 36
UPPER BODY / FULL BODY

- Frequency: 3-5 times/ week
- *Habits Rule You – Period 3 – Upper Body/Full Body* VIDEO

ACTIVE REST 1
Week 37 & 38

- Frequency: 3-6 times/week
- Leisure sports and activities

PERIOD 4
Week 39 – Week 50
UPPER & LOWER BODY

- Frequency: 4-6 times/ week
- Alternate between:

Habits Rule You – Period 4 – Upper Body VIDEO
&
Habits Rule You – Period 4 – Lower Body VIDEO

ACTIVE REST 2
Week 51 & 52

- Frequency: 3-5 times/week
- Leisure sports and activities

Working Out at the Gym

All that being said, if you wish to go to the gym instead of working out at home, once again, it is best to plan the year ahead. When it comes to working out at the gym many people don't really know how to work out correctly. Copying what others do could be helpful; however, in many instances it could be harmful if the person you're copying performs the exercise incorrectly.

Gym memberships should include a complimentary orientation, which is the perfect time to get yourself accustomed to the fitness equipment in the gym. During this orientation ask as many questions as you can about how the equipment works (take notes even), ask if they have a circuit area where the equipment is placed in a set order so that you could easily get a total body workout. In our gym, Giuseppe created a circuit area where the equipment was placed strategically so that members would get a full body workout by the time they completed the circuit. They could just hop from one machine to the next and by the time they were done, they equally hit all their muscle groups. Many gyms now have a designated area for circuit training.

When working out at the gym there are a few aspects to keep in mind, which apply when you also work out at home:
- Intensity
- Weight
- Breathing
- Range of Motion
- Technique
- Speed

Intensity

If your goal is to lose weight, pay attention to the intensity at which you work out. In order to lose fat— not muscle or water— the best approach is to work out at a moderate intensity. Generally, people think of cardio as means to lose weight, which is correct. However, some wrongfully assume that the higher the intensity the more calories are burnt, resulting in more weight loss. While high intensity cardio does burn more calories, the fat you think you're losing will actually not go away much. Instead, it's the particular muscles used in that cardio activity that get most of the workout. That will eventually translate into a bulkier body, simply because the fat will not be used as a fuel source with this type of training method.

When you're on a treadmill running at a *moderate* intensity, after a specific time (which is dictated by your particular fitness level) your body will kick into the *aerobic fuel system*. The aerobic system is a window in which the body has enough time to dig into your existing fat store and use them as fuel for the workout. The longer you stay at this level, the more fat you lose. In order to achieve this, cardio should be done at a moderate intensity— *your* moderate level, to be more specific. One way to find your ideal fat burning zone is by using this formula: first, figure out your maximum heart rate (220 minus your age). Your fat burning zone is 60%–70% of your maximum heart rate. So let's say you're 48 years old:

220 − 48 = 172
172 × 60% = 103.2
172 × 70% = 120.4

Your fat burning zone is when your heart beats 103 to 120 times per minute (or 17 to 20 beats per 10 seconds).

Another quick way to find out if you're in the fat burning zone is by making sure work out *hard enough to break a sweat, yet you're able to carry a conversation without gasping for air.*

The time it takes your body to kick into the aerobic system depends on your personal aerobic fitness level; the more fit you become, the faster the body moves into the fat burning zone, sometimes taking only minutes. So if you're a beginner at this, you have to be patient and keep working out at your moderate fitness level. By doing this, your body will start burning fat sooner and sooner. The more fit you become, the sooner your body will kick into the fat burning zone.

On the other hand, if you go past the moderate intensity over to high, your body switches to the *anaerobic fuel system*. While in this system, your body will need fuel at a much faster rate in order to fulfill the high demands of the workout. The body's fastest way to provide energy for an anaerobic workout is to use glucose. As glucose is the primary fuel source for the brain, you might be left feeling depleted or weak after an overly intense workout. This type of workout is used mainly by athletes, with the goal to increase strength, power, and build muscle mass.

To recap, if fat loss is your goal, keep your cardio at moderate intensity. As your fitness level improves, your moderate level will go up as well. The intensity at which you started working out will become lighter, so you'll have to gradually increase your intensity level as your endurance level rises.

Remember, you can always adjust yourself to keep it within the fat burning zone by making sure you *break a sweat, yet are able to carry a conversation without gasping for air.*

Weight

Regular strength training (3 to 5 times per week) improves muscle tone, strength, and helps increase bone density. Unlike a cardio routine where you want to keep it at moderate intensity in order to lose weight, here you want to push into your anaerobic energy system (I recommend doing this after you've completed Period 2, when you feel your strength had improved).

Lifting heavier weights at lower repetitions will give you more muscle tone and definition. I heard many women being reluctant to lift heavy weights, thinking they will build muscles and bulk up. That is not something to worry about because, as women, we don't have the adequate testosterone levels to build that kind of muscular volume; you'd have to be on a very specific, intensive bodybuilding program to become very muscular.

The good news about building muscle tone is that your toned muscles act like an engine, needing energy 24 hours a day. In other words, while you're sleeping at night or are simply resting, your muscles are feasting on the existing fat stores to get their energy needs. This translates into fat loss which, in my opinion, makes strength training one of the best ways to lose fat.

An important aspect to keep in mind, particularly when lifting heavier weights, is to stretch at the end of each session. This gives your muscles time to relax back into their previous length. If you don't stretch, the increase in muscle tone will actually lead to a reduced range of motion. This can cause interesting inconveniences (such as not being able to lift or twist your arms as before), and in some cases even injuries. There were a few massive guys at the gym, who used to do their weight training routines religiously. But when it came to stretching, they didn't think it was that important. As a result, the range of motion in their shoulders was so drastically reduced, in order to get rid of an itch on their back they needed assistance from each other! Now following a normal strength training routine will not cause you to not be able to scratch your own back, but you get my point as to the importance of stretching.

Breathing

Particularly when lifting weights, how you breathe becomes very important. Make sure you breathe *out* when you go against gravity, so that you don't build pressure in your chest and possibly pass out. For example, when you do bicep curls, breathe out while lifting the weights, and breathe in during the downward motion.

Range of Motion

Make sure to complete each exercise using full range of motion. Keep the muscles always under tension and most importantly, on the downward motion (called the *eccentric* phase) control the weights as much as you would in the upward motion.

Technique

Never rest the weight on locked joints. When lifting weights, always keep joints slightly bent and stop the motion just before the joint locks. Locking eventually causes injuries, especially if using heavier weights. Try to go through your entire range of motion, but do not lock your joints.

Speed

Better results are achieved when you don't rush. The effectiveness of the exercise increases substantially when you control the movement and actually take longer, particularly through the second part of the exercise called the eccentric phase. A rule of thumb is using the 2:3 ratio: 2 seconds on the way up (when going against gravity) and 3 seconds on the way down.

The following is your one-year plan explained.

Period 1 (12 weeks)

For this first period I would advise to start with a light whole-body circuit training using selectorized equipment, to get your muscles and tendons accustomed to the new activity (remember your adaption phase). Again, make sure you attend the orientation at your gym and ask as many questions as you need in order to understand how to properly use the equipment, so that you prevent any injuries. Ask particularly if there is a circuit training area where you can get a total body workout.

I wouldn't suggest using free weights for this period, especially if this is your first time working out. Using free weights requires that you have an already toned core and enough knowledge in executing the exercises properly. If used incorrectly, free weights can pull your body out of alignment, which can possibly result in injuries. The selectorized equipment is safer due to its fixed nature.

Do not take this period lightly. You might feel like you could do more, but your tendons don't. Skipping or rushing through this period of adaptation by raising the intensity might cause joint and muscle discomfort, as well as injuries down the road.

If weight loss is your goal, don't take breaks in between your sets; go from one piece of equipment to the next, making sure you use low weights but high repetitions of 15 to 20. If you can only do 10 repetitions (instead of 15-20), you know the weight is too heavy for this type of workout, so lower the weight. On the other hand, if the weight allows you to do 30 reps, then you should increase the weight. The last couple of repetitions should be hard to complete but you should keep going and push through—the last few repetitions are the ones that make change happen.

Once you've completed the circuit, quickly hop on a cardio machine (elliptical, treadmill, rower, etc) for 5- 15 minutes. If time and endurance allow, go back to the circuit area and start all over again.

Try to consistently keep your heart rate up at a moderate level: make sure you break a sweat but are still able to carry a conversation without gasping for air.

Period 2 (12 weeks)

For this period, you can continue focusing on your whole body, just in a different way. Consider taking a few different aerobic classes that use free weights, and mix them up with classes that are sports related, such as boxing and kickboxing. Remember, best results are achieved when you surprise your body with a different routine. You had just finished doing total body conditioning for 3 months; now it's time to change your routine to one that targets those muscles more intensely and in a different way.

Period 3 (12 weeks)

For this period go back on the selectorized equipment. This time you want to do strength training and cardio separately.

For the strength training portion, expand by using the rest of the selectorized equipment on the gym floor, as well as free weights. Just make sure you use the free weights correctly. At this point, it's worth purchasing a session with a facility instructor to get proper instruction as to how to correctly use free weights in order to avoid injuries and get better results. To give you a few points here, you should always remember to keep your spine and neck straight, and not hyperextend or lock your joints.

For this period divide the main muscle groups into 2 separate workouts, and work them out alternatively. If you decide to work out 4 times per week, alternate the 2 different workouts. This way you hit the same muscle group twice a week. An example would be:

- Strength training 1 (Monday & Wednesday): chest, quads, biceps, outer thigh, middle shoulders, glutes, low back, obliques.
- Strength training 2 (Tuesday & Thursday): back (lats), hamstrings, triceps, inner thigh, front shoulders, calves, abs, rear shoulders.

You can always add an extra day or 2 to your weekly program if you choose to, only make sure you never work out the same muscle group 2 days in a row. With the exception of abs, all muscles need 48 hours to fully recover from strength training. For example:

- Strength training 1 (Monday, Wednesday & Friday): chest, quads, biceps, outer thigh, middle shoulders, glutes, low back, obliques.

- Strength training 2 (Tuesday, Thursday & Saturday): back (lats), hamstrings, triceps, inner thigh, front shoulders, calves, abs, rear shoulders.

During Period 3, you should push it a bit more by increasing your weights and lowering the repetitions—anywhere between 8 to 10 repetitions is the rule of thumb. The last couple of reps should be difficult to lift, but push to complete the set. If you can do more than 10 repetitions, it means the weight is too light, so increase it (again, ladies, don't worry about lifting heavy weights; you won't bulk up).

Depending on how much time you have available, do each set 2 or 3 times in a row. Take 40 – 60 second breaks in between sets. Use this time to stretch, to release some of the tension and avoid a decrease in range of motion.

This type of workout is more demanding and helps increase your muscle tone, mass, and strength. Stretching becomes even more so important at this point, so incorporate it with your training. Between sets and while you walk from one piece of equipment to the next, lightly stretch the muscles you just worked out to release some of the tension and avoid a decrease in your range of motion. The stretch also becomes more effective because your muscles are warm at this point.

Once you're done your strength training portion of your program (anywhere between 30-40 minutes), hop on the treadmill, elliptical, rower, bike, etc, for your cardio portion (roughly 30 minutes should be fine). You could also do your cardio by jogging to and from the gym, and get fresh air in the process. That being said, indoor cardio equipment comes in handy when the weather is unfavorable.

Active rest 1 (2 weeks)

Both periods 3 and 4 are more intense, so now you need to give your body a chance to recover before you go on the last period. Aside from playing sports, going hiking and bike riding, you could take advantage of some of the other programs and classes offered at the gym, such as yoga, Pilates, swimming, badminton, dance, etc.

Period 4 (12 weeks)

In Period 3, you pushed your muscles to expand more. Now you want them to retain their shape, while increasing their density. Improving the density of your muscles is something you ultimately want to achieve. When muscle fibers get denser, the muscles maintain their tone for a longer period of time. Then if for some reason you stop lifting weights for a while, it will take longer to lose muscle tone. And when you resume your strength training program, your muscles will spring back into shape much quicker.

You can follow a similar split routine as in Period 3, plus make the following adjustments:

- Lower the weights to a minimum (even 5 lbs), and increase your repetitions to a maximum (anywhere from 25 all the way up to 50 and even 75). This should be applied to all muscle groups, from chest and back, to inner and outer thigh muscles. It might sound like a waste of time to be doing so many repetitions, but when you actually do it, you'll realize the amazing benefits this type of workout gives. I

particularly favor it because it kind of sets in place all the previous hard work and truly defines the body.
- Do not take breaks in between sets. This adds a cardio aspect to the workout. Because this type of workout combines both strength and cardio, it helps reduce stubborn intramuscular fat (or visceral fat), which is what in the end gives your muscles great definition.

Active rest (2 weeks)

For your active rest, again, choose from classes and programs offered at the gym such as yoga, Pilates, swimming, badminton, dance, etc.

WORKING OUT AT THE GYM
One-Year Fitness Chart

PERIOD 1
Week 1 – Week 12
FULL BODY CIRCUIT

- Frequency: 3 times/week
- Type of Training: Full Body Circuit
- Weights: Low–Moderate
- Repetitions: Moderate (15–20)
- Number of Sets: 1 set each exercise
- No breaks in between sets
- Add Cardio 2–3 other days of the week

Full Body Circuit on selectorized equipment, 1 set each exercise. After you hit all your muscle groups once, hop on a piece of cardio equipment for 5–15 minutes (treadmill, rowing machine, elliptical, etc). Repeat this cycle for as long as your time allows.

PERIOD 2
Week 13 – Week 24
FULL BODY

- Frequency: 3–5 times/ week
- Type of Training: Mix Aerobic Classes

Aerobic Classes containing Strength Training and Sports related Classes such as Boxing & Kickboxing

PERIOD 3

Week 25 – Week 36
FULL BODY

- Frequency: 4-6 times/ week
- Type of Training: Strength & Cardio/Endurance (Separate)
- Weights: High
- Repetitions: Low (8-12)
- Number of Sets: 2-3 each exercise
- 40-60 sec. breaks in between sets

Strength Training: Selectorized Equipment & Free weights
Cardio Training: Elliptical, Treadmill, Rowing machine, etc.

Monday & Wednesday – Strength Training 1:

Back 2-3 sets, 8 – 12 reps
Biceps 2-3 sets, 8 – 12 reps
Rear shoulders 2-3 sets, 8 – 12 reps
Low back 2-3 sets, 8 – 12 reps
Chest 2-3 sets, 8 – 12 reps
Triceps 2-3 sets, 8 – 12 reps
Front shoulders 2-3 sets, 8 – 12 reps
Abs 2-3 sets, 8 – 12 reps
Middle shoulders 2-3 sets, 8 – 12 reps
Cardio: Roughly 30 minutes (or jog home)

Tuesday & Thursday (and/or Friday) – Strength Training 2:

Quads 2-3 sets, 8 – 12 reps
Hamstrings 2-3 sets, 8 – 12 reps
Calves 2-3 sets, 8 – 10 reps
Inner thigh 2-3 sets, 8 – 12 reps
Outer thigh 2-3 sets, 8 – 12 reps
Glutes 2-3 sets, 8 – 12 reps
Right Obliques 2-3 sets, 8 – 12 reps
Left Obliques 2-3 sets, 8 – 12 reps
Cardio: Roughly 30 minutes (or jog home)

ACTIVE REST 1
Week 37 & Week 38
- Frequency: 4-6 times/week
Classes (Yoga, Pilates, Dance, etc)

PERIOD 4
Week 39 - Week 50
FULL BODY

- Frequency: 4-6 times/ week
- Type of Training: Muscle Definition
- Weights: Low
- Repetitions: High (25-50-75)
- Number of Sets: 1 set each exercise
- No breaks in between sets
- Selectorized equipment & Free weights
- Cardio training: Elliptical, treadmill, rowing machine, etc

Monday & Wednesday - Strength training 1:

Back 1 set, 25 - 50 - 75 reps
Biceps 1 set, 25 - 50 - 75 reps
Rear shoulders 1 set, 25 - 50 - 75 reps
Low back 1 set, 25 - 50 - 75 reps
Chest 1 set, 25 - 50 - 75 reps
Triceps 1 set, 25 - 50 - 75 reps
Front shoulders 1 set, 25 - 50 - 75 reps
Abs 1 set, 25 - 50 - 75 reps
Middle shoulders 1 set, 25 - 50 - 75 reps
Cardio: roughly 30 minutes (or jog home)

Tuesday & Thursday (and/or Friday) - Strength training 2:

Quads 1 set, 25 - 50 - 75 reps
Hamstrings 1 set, 25 - 50 - 75 reps
Calves 1 set, 25 - 50 - 75 reps
Inner thigh 1 set, 25 - 50 - 75 reps
Outer thigh 1 set, 25 - 50 - 75 reps
Glutes 1 set, 25 - 50 - 75 reps
Right Obliques 1 set, 25 - 50 - 75 reps
Left Obliques 1 set, 25 - 50 - 75 reps
Cardio: roughly 30 minutes (or jog home)

ACTIVE REST 2

Week 51 & Week 52
Frequency: 4-6 times/week

Classes (Yoga, Pilates, Dance, etc)

HIRING A PERSONAL TRAINER

You're a buzzing bee at home, you take your walks, power walks or runs regularly, and you follow a generalized workout routine at home or at the gym. You created a set of beautiful, life-promoting habits which improved— if not prolonged— your life. Now you're contemplating taking it to the next level by hiring a personal trainer. This is the ideal time to do so, as your tendons, muscles and cardiovascular systems are conditioned enough to be safely pushed to the next level of intensity.

Hiring a personal trainer is the best way to take your fitness to the next level. Just be aware of the ones that have their ears plugged to your concerns. There are personal trainers who got certified after taking a 2-weekend course, and there are personal trainers who went to college or university and studied for many years. How do you know which one to put your trust in? One thing I learned in this business is that a beautifully framed certification hung on the wall doesn't always imply common sense or guarantee compassion for their clients. A certification doesn't weight much, unless the personal trainer continuously keeps up with the newest research. Fitness is a fairly new field in which new discoveries are still being made; there are exercises that used to be taught 20 or 10 or even 5 years ago, which today are considered outlawed because they put strain on the body and lead to injuries. Obviously, if your trainer went to school 20 years ago and never opened another book since, you might have a problem. On the other hand, a personal trainer who just got out of school, although not experienced, might be better educated in the latest training techniques.

A good personal trainer does not work on templates. A good personal trainer does not put you in a box, train you the same as they would the rest of their clients. A good personal trainer puts you in your own category. He or she will not only thoroughly assess your fitness level, but they will take into consideration your past and present injuries, the kind of job you do, what habits you have at home, etc. *"No pain no gain"* doesn't apply indiscriminately to all cases— if you have an injury that screams out when you do your push-ups, YOU SHOULD STOP. I heard trainers shout at their clients "Keep going, no pain no gain", which in this particular case is the epitome of ignorance. Don't assume that if someone is certified in training the human body, he or she knows what they're doing. Interview your potential trainer. Ask to see before and after pictures, ideally even talk to their clients. There are a few important questions you'd want to ask: "Did you get the results you expected or at least close to what you expected?", and "How does your body feel compared to before you started training: did your past aches and pains subside, do you have the same, or did you get new ones?" Yes, you want to get results in your appearance, but most importantly, you want to feel better than before.

Once you made your decision, let your personal trainer know of your year-long plan; ask that he or she guides you to properly integrate their custom routine into your program. Always remember to keep up with your stretches, especially at the end of the day.

Afterword

Everything I was taught, plus the things I discovered myself along the way by simply living and learning, I was applying in my life and finally started feeling like myself again— I regained my energy, my strength, and my emotional balance. So technically, I didn't need to put it in a book.

However, when we come to learn something valuable, we can't just keep it all to ourselves thinking it's all good— it doesn't work that way. You, and I, and everybody else, are responsible to share the useful information we came to learn and help others.

Did you hear of the *One hundredth monkey effect*? It goes like this: ninety-nine monkeys learned a new behavior of washing their sweet potatoes in a stream before eating. As soon as the hundredth monkey adopted this behavior (the numbers not to be taken literally), this behavior spread through "thin air" on the other side of the sea— other monkey tribes started doing the same thing. That one extra monkey was what it took to keep the momentum going, and set the idea of the new behavior in motion over to a distant place. That *one* extra monkey made the change possible.

Undeniably, there is something connecting all life— a powerful force that bypasses distance, time, and space. Then it dawned on me that our little universe might not be as little as we think; that it might include more than just our loved ones. When we feel better, people living in the most remote corners of the world feel it. They may not know it, but they can feel it. So when we make the decision to take care of ourselves, others may be inspired to do the same for themselves. And that makes us collectively responsible for the well-being of each other. You don't know if you are in the position of that hundredth monkey, the one that will actually cause the change. But you are one extra person who can help keep it all in motion, move it forward, encourage others to do the same; so that we collectively tip the scale toward beauty. You might think this is corny but— and I say this as lovingly as I possibly can— I really don't care what you think, if what you think is in the slightest way unhelpful. I say the world needs more "corny" today than ever before.

Countless hours of work go into the making of beautiful films, documentaries and books, emphasizing the importance of each of us. Still, too many don't take it literally. We might even shed a little tear while watching a beautiful film, but once the movie ends, we shake ourselves of the "illusion" and carry on with our old habitual routines.

So here is where I'm proposing to start: we're going to start with taking beautiful things literally. In order to be willing to put in the work and be successful at creating better habits it's imperative to understand that you are one hundred percent worth it. We are going to start with the reality that you are valuable and that every single person in this world needs you. IT'S A DONE DEAL. That is our starting point. You might consider this notion farfetched, but remember the hundredth monkey effect I talked about earlier. Every one of your choices has implications that don't stop at the person you see when you look in the mirror. You hold a much broader scope— to lift yourself, and others along with you. Your emotional wellbeing, your level of contentment, of joy, your daring to reach for remarkable dreams without letting setbacks slow you down, your overcoming negative habits one at a time... all this affects not only you and the people close to you. You can be that *one* extra person that is ultimately needed to make the change possible at the big level. Create constructive habits that bring you up and you can help salvage the world. SEE HOW PRECIOUS YOU ARE? This preciousness— although we have the freedom to delay believing as long as we wish— can never be altered.

There are countless possibilities laying ahead. Things can change, but you have to make the decision to set them in motion and stick to it. Stop looking back counting your "failures" or you'll fall off the path, crash into that stubborn oak tree standing by the side of the road and add yet another disappointment to your resume. Look ahead, focus on the possibility. Look forward with hope, because even though we are not able to change past mistakes or "failures", they are not permanent. The Greek philosopher Heraclitus said, "*There is nothing permanent except change.*" Nothing is permanent— no sickness, no anxiety, no nightmares or betrayal. None of these will stay the way they are forever. Nothing is permanent but God, Who made you. Therefore, you and your flawlessness are permanent— *it's in your nature*. That means that you're "stuck" with yourself for a very long time. So you might as well start believing it, you might as well start acting upon it.

How do you do that? By focusing your attention on your brain, the place where habits are developed. How you make use of your brain— what you choose to focus on in every moment— creates your everyday habits, which in turn create your emotions, which in turn influence your actions. So next time you catch yourself doubting or procrastinating, next time you feel guilty, irritated, angry, powerless or discouraged, know that in doing so you're strengthening a habit that only reinforces all those feelings. It's ok to feel negative emotions, but only to be used as a tool to steer yourself in the right direction. The fastest way to find out if you're in a good habit-creating mode is by assessing how you feel. When you focus on thinking *beautiful,* you feel good. And by being consistent in doing so, more *beautiful* will come back via habits.

Create a new positive habit today: be mindful of your thoughts, especially of your recurring ones. The habit of negative internalizing— one I mentioned in the introduction as the most devious of all— not only makes you feel dreadful on its own, but it can become the root of other negative habits such as overeating, smoking, even drug abuse.

Whether we do it consciously or by default, each of us is responsible of the habits we create. You can make a habit of believing in your inner voice telling you of the great potential you hold, or you can make a habit of opening your ears to statistics shoved in your face by the "peanut gallery" and let your dream be crushed before it sees the light of day. Which scenario do you choose? It's as simple as that.

Nothing defines us more than our habits. Everything that we do— from what we eat and how much we eat, to how we move, how we talk, what we believe in, even the way we cross our arms— are the result of habits; how we perceive life around us, whether we allow stress to get the best of us, if we are generally more positive or negative, even our characters, are all results of habits created over a period of time. Whether we want it or not, whether we even accept it or not, our habits— good *and* bad— rule us. It seems we have no choice but to be creatures of habits.

So why not turn that in your favor? Why not create life-promoting habits— the kind that bring out your true identity, your true self? You can let habits create by default, or you can take control and bring to life some beautiful things purposely— your choice. Let your default mechanism take over and it will easily generate unanswered questions for you. Use it as a tool, and you will feel the freedom of coming into your own. Your positive habits bring out the vastness in you. Your negative habits on the other hand, conceal it by creating a mask. This mask is a lie that works against you. That being said, who you truly are underneath has nothing to do with the image you show of yourself via your bad habits. So what are your habits? Who are you in this moment? Are you showing your true self, or are you showing a lie?

Life is precious. Even though it's eternal— we do have "all the time in the world"— it would be a shame not to take a proactive step and live it fully today. So GET UP! So what if you don't succeed the first time? So what if you don't succeed the second, third or even tenth time? Don't worry about how long it takes to get there. How long did it take you, or any of us for that matter, to become the complex beings that we are? *"Practice makes perfect"*, which is exactly what we've all been doing. You might not see your goal fully realized yet, but you succeeded in something equally as valuable: you learned what *doesn't work*. Next time you attempt to do it again you'll be smarter, more prepared, wiser, and most definitely closer to your goal. And if you happen to fall, simply get up— yes, again— and continue what you started. Know that with each and every time you consciously switch your focus on your goal, you are getting closer to it.

Anyone can break free from the vicious circle of playing hide-and-seek with their life's purpose; age should never be a factor. Both a 15 and an 80-year old could be successful at creating life-promoting habits if they choose to. Listen to the right voice inside of you, the one that never deceives. Allow it to have the last word. No matter how old, no matter how talentless or insignificant you may think you are, the right voice inside of you is much stronger than the image you have of yourself. The right voice inside of you will always see you as the most elegant, most beautiful, creative human being, simply because you are. Those qualities are very much real and so your dreams and goals are perfectly attainable. They are attainable because *you are your dreams, you are your goals*. You dream of them because that is your true identity.

Now, with this kind of mentality, reaching for your desired weight, health goal, your dream job or passion, become exciting possibilities. Because you have the confidence that is solely up to you to make it real. It is solely in your power to ditch the negative habits and create life-promoting ones.

To find out what your hindering habitual behaviors are, perform an honest assessment of your existing habits. Then do whatever it takes to stop falling prey to their short-lived rewards. Learning what it is that has been keeping you from becoming the best version of you is possibly one of the most valuable pieces of information you could learn about yourself. Think of habits in the form of repetitive actions, to habits of thought in the form of general ideas and beliefs. Think of your health, your emotions, your relationships, think of your goals. Figure out what you want, then think of creating new, life-promoting habits that will support it— from habits of *doing* what's right, to habits of *thinking* what's right. Always remember this: whatever your goal is, it's DONE— your goal is alive and well, and it's waiting for you. Pursue it with confidence now, knowing that with every ounce of persistence and patience that you have you are getting closer to it.

Yes, there are going to be "failures" and yes, there are going to be challenging people trying hard (sometimes *very* hard) to steer you away from your heart. But always remember that both— failures and unsupportive people— are only there to make you stronger. They push you into going back to the drawing board and *think.* They are there to teach you of who you really are and to stay focused on what you want. This is the kind of habitual mentality that turns a seemingly permanent failure into a stepping-stone.

Lastly, something I cannot emphasize enough: being fearless is vital. There is always a positive outcome when we *wake up* from our own fears and live truthful to our inherent potential. Being fearless is the key to having clarity, allows one to expand and grow, it gives freedom to think outside the box and dare to birth outstanding dreams. Being fearless is what you need to be in order to fully liberate your potential.

I'm not going to stay here and tell you "anything is possible" but what I am going to tell you is this: *never give up on yourself.* No matter where you are on this planet, no matter the conditions around you, it can always get better if you choose it to be better. It can always get better if you choose to adopt a positive perspective and appreciate everything that makes up your moment of *now*. It can always get better if you choose to hold on to the *possibility*, instead of the thought of not wanting to be where you are. It can always get better if you focus on the clear picture of what you want to achieve, if you stay strong and persistent. It can always get better if you stay loyal to the truth inside, if you follow your heart. Only then are limiting boundaries and man-made rules broken. Only then does *"anything is possible"* become more than just words, as you will feel their meaning and naturally live it.

Starting NOW, give it a year. Don't wait until you get the perfect pair of runners or the right sports bra, don't wait for the first of the month, and definitely don't wait for the New Year. I mentioned this earlier and I'm mentioning it again because it's extremely important to know what actually happens when you do that— it means that you're not ready to start at all. When you're hesitant about starting and happen to "cheat" or miss a workout (for example), chances are you'll think the whole thing is ruined, and that in order to make it work you have to start everything all over. But that's not true. Your results may be delayed but they are most definitely not ruined. The work you put in so far— no matter how little— is already in the bank, so to speak. So pick yourself up and continue what you had already started. Think simple, stay focused, be persistent, be patient.

One morning you'll wake up and be amazed at what you've accomplished.

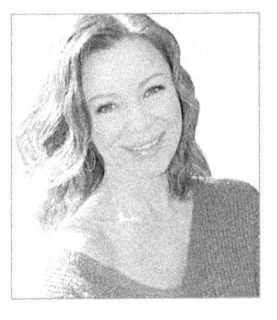

Angelica Ganea is the recipient of the *Award of Excellence* from CanPak Chamber of Commerce Canada, for breaking cultural barriers through singing. She is also the author of 'Remember Who You Are: the Story Behind the Song', a book which accompanies her original music CD.

Habits Rule You: One Simple Answer to Achieving Your Nutrition & Fitness Goals is the first book in Angelica Ganea's series of self-help works.

CREATE POSITIVE EATING & EXERCISING HABITS WITH ANGELICA'S PERSONALIZED 1 YEAR PLAN

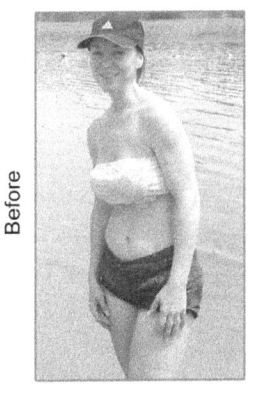

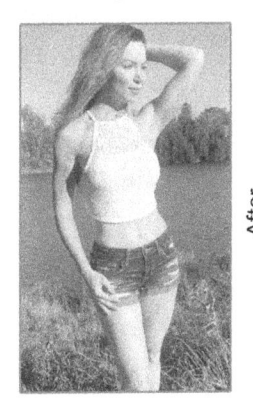

Before

After

FOR INFORMATION ON PROGRAMS VISIT
www.HabitsRuleYou.com

To get your access code to Angelica's complimentary fitness videos, please visit

www.AngelicaGanea.com/videos.html

CPSIA information can be obtained
at www.ICGtesting.com
Printed in the USA
LVHW030549070220
646151LV00001B/8